Essentials in Ophthalmology

Vitreo-retinal Surgery

B. Kirchhof   D. Wong
Editors

Essentials in Ophthalmology

G. K. Krieglstein   R. N. Weinreb
Series Editors

Glaucoma

Cataract and Refractive Surgery

Uveitis and Immunological Disorders

Vitreo-retinal Surgery

Medical Retina

Oculoplastics and Orbit

Pediatric Ophthalmology,
Neuro-Ophthalmology, Genetics

Cornea and External Eye Disease

Editors   Bernd Kirchhof
David Wong

Vitreo-retinal Surgery

With 122 Figures, Mostly in Colour
and 13 Tables

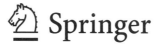 Springer

Series Editors

Günter K. Krieglstein, MD
Professor and Chairman
Department of Ophthalmology
University of Cologne
Kerpener Straße 62
50924 Cologne
Germany

Robert N. Weinreb, MD
Professor and Director
Hamilton Glaucoma Center
Department of Ophthalmology
University of California at San Diego
9500 Gilman Drive
La Jolla, CA 92093-0946
USA

Volume Editors

Bernd Kirchhof, MD
Professor and Chairman
Department of Vitreo-retinal Surgery
Center for Ophthalmology
University of Cologne
Kerpener Straße 62
50924 Cologne
Germany

David Wong, MD
Professor and Chairman
Department of Ophthalmology
Faculty of Medicine
University of Hong Kong
21 Sassoon Road, Pok Fu Lam
Hong Kong

ISBN-10   3-540-33669-9
Springer Berlin Heidelberg NewYork

ISBN-13   978-3-540-33669-3
Springer Berlin Heidelberg NewYork

ISSN 1612-3212

Library of Congress Control Number: 2006935425

Springer is a part of Springer Science + Business Media

springer.com

The use of general descriptive names, registered names, trademarks, etc. in this publication does not imply, even in the absence of a specific statement, that such names are exempt from the relevant protective laws and regulations and therefore free for general use.

Product liability: The publishers cannot guarantee the accuracy of any information about dosage and application contained in this book. In every individual case the user must check such information by consulting the relevant literature.

Editor: Marion Philipp, Heidelberg, Germany
Desk Editor: Martina Himberger, Heidelberg, Germany
Production: LE-TeX Jelonek, Schmidt & Vöckler GbR, Leipzig, Germany
Cover Design: Erich Kirchner, Heidelberg, Germany

Printed on acid-free paper
24/3100Wa   5 4 3 2 1 0

Foreword

The series *Essentials in Ophthalmology* was initiated two years ago to expedite the timely transfer of new information in vision science and evidence-based medicine into clinical practice. We thought that this prospicient idea would be moved and guided by a resolute commitment to excellence. It is reasonable to now update our readers with what has been achieved.

The immediate goal was to transfer information through a high quality quarterly publication in which ophthalmology would be represented by eight subspecialties. In this regard, each issue has had a subspecialty theme and has been overseen by two internationally recognized volume editors, who in turn have invited a bevy of experts to discuss clinically relevant and appropriate topics. Summaries of clinically relevant information have been provided throughout each chapter.

Each subspecialty area now has been covered once, and the response to the first eight volumes in the series has been enthusiastically positive. With the start of the second cycle of subspecialty coverage, the dissemination of practical information will be continued as we learn more about the emerging advances in various ophthalmic subspecialties that can be applied to obtain the best possible care of our patients. Moreover, we will continue to highlight clinically relevant information and maintain our commitment to excellence.

G. K. Krieglstein
R. N. Weinreb
Series Editors

Preface

This second edition promises to challenge our ideas about vitreoretinal surgery. As expected, some new and innovative techniques are described, the most exciting of which is the use of free retinal pigment epithelium patch grafts in patients with atrophic macular degeneration. We are interested in the advances that have made this surgery possible and look forward to the long-term outcomes. In the last couple of years, surgeons have become increasingly convinced by the advantages conferred by smaller gauge instruments, brighter and even safer lights, combined with an innovative viewing system to make routine surgery quicker and less traumatic for the patients. The use of 25-gauge for tumor biopsies is an exciting new development that represents a huge advantage over needle biopsies. The indication and the rationale for biopsies in cases of suspected uveal melanoma are presented.

There will always of course be difficult clinical decisions; choices have to be made despite the absence of good data based on randomized trials. A good example of a dilemma is whether to perform early vitrectomy for postoperative endophthalmitis. For this edition, we have opposing views from two surgeons. You simply have to read and decide for yourself. There are other controversies such as vitrectomy for floaters: the preparation in terms of counseling, patient selection, and pitfalls are well covered in a chapter on the subject.

The chapter on macular holes examines the evidence behind our current practice. Despite the high success rate, a minority of patients will fail to respond to conventional surgery and a novel approach with heavy silicone oil is presented.

Sometimes, the skill of a surgeon is to know when not to operate. Asymptomatic inferior retinal detachment is another controversial area explored in a reasoned fashion, though no one knows for sure the cause of optical coherence tomography findings of subclinical macular retinal detachments.

Then we come to the big topic of tamponading. The need to apply scleral buckling, to adopt postoperative head-down posturing, or to use long-acting gas for inferior retinal breaks are being challenged as more rhegmatogenous retinal detachments are treated using primary vitrectomy and air alone. There is renewed interest in the techniques for draining subretinal fluid and the chapter on slippage explains how unwanted retinal folds can be avoided, whilst offering an easy technique for the exchange of fluids and the injection of silicone oil.

We hope you will enjoy reading this book as much as we have preparing it.

Bernd Kirchhof
David Wong
Editors

Contents

Chapter 4
**Slippage of the Retina: What Causes
It and How Can It Be Prevented?**

David Wong

Chapter 5
**Complete and Early Vitrectomy
for Endophthalmitis (CEVE)
as Today's Alternative to the
Endophthalmitis Vitrectomy Study**

Ferenc Kuhn, Giampaolo Gini

Chapter 6

**Treatment of Acute Bacterial
Endophthalmitis After Cataract
Surgery Without Vitrectomy**

Thomas Theelen, Maurits A.D. Tilanus

Chapter 7

New Instruments in Vitrectomy

Masahito Ohji, Yasuo Tano

Chapter 8

25-Gauge Biopsy of Uveal Tumors

Bertil Damato, Carl Groenewald

Chapter 9
Vitrectomy Against Floaters

Hans Hoerauf

Chapter 10
Treatment of Retinal Detachment from Inferior Breaks with Pars Plana Vitrectomy

Vicente Martinez-Castillo, Jose Garcia-Arumi, Anna Boixadera, Miguel A. Zapata

Chapter 11
Subclinical Retinal Detachment

Jose Garcia-Arumi, Anna Boixadera, Vicente
Martinez-Castillo, Miguel A. Zapata

Chapter 12
**Autologous Translocation
of the Choroid and RPE in Patients
with Geographic Atrophy**

Antonia M. Joussen, Jan van Meurs, Bernd
Kirchhof

Contributors

James Bainbridge
Moorfields Eye Hospital
City Road
London EC1V 2PD
UK

Anna Boixadera
Hospital Vall d´ Hebron
Servicio de Oftalmologia
Paseo Vall d´ Hebron, 119 – 121
Barcelona
Spain

David G. Charteris
Moorfields Eye Hospital
City Road
London EC1V 2PD
UK

Bertil Damato
Royal Liverpool University Hospital
Prescot Street
Liverpool L7 8XP
UK

Jose Garcia-Arumi
Instituto de Microcirugía Ocular
C/ Munner n° 10
08022 Barcelona
Spain

Giampaolo Gini
City Hospital
Viale Vittorio Veneto 60
Prato 59100
Italy

Zdenek Gregor
Moorfields Eye Hospital
City Road
London EC1V 2PD
UK

Carl Groenewald
Royal Liverpool University Hospital
Prescot Street
Liverpool L7 8XP
UK

Hans Hoerauf
University Eye Clinic, UK S-H
Campus Lübeck
Lübeck
Germany

Antonia M. Joussen
Department of Ophthalmology
University of Duesseldorf
Moorenstraße 5
40225 Duesseldorf
Germany

Bernd Kirchhof
Department of Vitreo-retinal Surgery
Center for Ophthalmology
University of Cologne
Kerpener Straße 62
50924 Cologne
Germany

Ferenc Kuhn
University of Alabama at Birmingham
1201 11th Avenue South, Suite 300
Birmingham
AL 35205
USA

Vicente Martínez-Castillo
Hospital Vall d´ Hebron
Servicio de Oftalmologia
Paseo Vall d´ Hebron, 119 – 121
Barcelona
Spain

Masahito Ohji
Shiga University of Medical Science
Osaka University Medical School, E-7
Department of Ophthalmology
2-2 Yamidaoka Suita
Osaka 565-0871
Japan

Stanislao Rizzo
Chirurgica Oftalmica Ospedale S. Chiara
Via Roma 55
56100 Pisa
Italy

Yasuo Tano
Shiga University of Medical Science
Osaka University Medical School, E-7
Department of Ophthalmology
2-2 Yamidaoka Suita
Osaka 565-0871
Japan

Thomas Theelen
Academish Ziekenhuis Nijmegen
Philips van Leydenlaan 15
6525 EX Nijmegen
The Netherlands

Maurits A.D. Tilanus
Academish Ziekenhuis Nijmegen
Philips van Leydenlaan 15
6525 EX Nijmegen
The Netherlands

Jan van Meurs
Rotterdam Eye Hospital
Postbus 70030
3000 LM Rotterdam
The Netherlands

David Wong
Department of Ophthalmology
Faculty of Medicine
University of Hong Kong
21 Sassoon Road, Pok Fu Lam
Hong Kong

Miguel A. Zapata
C/ Sta Teresa 70 2º 1ª
08172 Sant Cugat
Spain

Chapter 1

Macular Holes

1

James Bainbridge, Zdenek Gregor

Core Messages

■ Idiopathic full-thickness macular holes are believed to result from tangential and antero-posterior traction exerted by the posterior vitreous cortex on the neurosensory retina at the fovea.

■ Only a minority of full-thickness macular holes resolve spontaneously and there is a significant risk of macular hole development in the fellow eye.

■ Surgical management by removal of the posterior cortical vitreous and long-acting intraocular gas tamponade results in a high rate of anatomical closure and a benefit to visual function.

■ Modifications to this surgical technique, proposed with the aim of improving anatomical and visual outcomes, include the use of adjuvants to stimulate glial repair and the dissection of the inner limiting membrane, with or without the aid of vital stains. The value of these modifications is not well-established.

■ The importance of prolonged face-down posturing to the rate of macular hole closure is unproven.

1.1 Epidemiology

A macular hole is a full-thickness defect of the neurosensory retina involving the anatomical fovea. Idiopathic full-thickness macular holes are an important cause of central visual loss; these lesions are twice as common in females as in males [1, 2] and three-quarters of affected individuals are over the age of 65 years [1]. The population prevalence of macular holes is estimated as being 0.1% in individuals aged 40 years or older and 0.8% in those aged over 74 years. No significant systemic risk factor for the development of macular holes has been identified although a possible association with the menopause has been described [1].

1.2 Pathogenesis

The pathogenesis of idiopathic full-thickness macular holes is not well understood. Macular holes are commonly idiopathic in etiology, although trauma and high myopia are implicated in a minority of cases. On the basis of clinical observations, ocular imaging, histological studies, and the results of vitrectomy surgery, the mechanism underlying idiopathic macular hole is widely believed to involve tangential as well as antero-posterior traction exerted by the posterior vitreous cortex on the neurosensory retina at the fovea. Evidence of the role of posterior vitreous attachment in the development of macular holes includes its association with an increased risk of macular hole development in the fellow eyes of individuals with unilateral macular holes and with the subsequent enlargement of established holes [3, 4]. There is no consensus on the exact mechanism of vitreo-foveal traction. Tangential traction may be the result of contraction of the prefoveal vitreous cortex following invasion and proliferation of Müller cells [5]. Anteroposterior traction may occur from dynamic tractional forces on an abnormally persistent vitreo-foveal attachment following perifoveal vitreous separation [6, 7]. The role of antero-posterior vitreo-foveal traction is supported by optical coherence tomography (OCT) studies that clearly identify perifoveal posterior hyaloid separation with persistent adherence of the posterior hyaloid to the centre of the fovea [6–8]. A cone-shaped zone of Müller cells, the 'Müller cell cone' forms the central and inner part of the fovea centralis and appears to confer structural support, serving as a plug to bind together the foveolar photoreceptor cells [9]. Vitreo-foveal traction may result in disinsertion of the Müller cell cone from underlying foveolar photoreceptor cells and in the formation of a foveal schisis or "cyst" [6–8]. A dehiscence develops in the roof of the foveal cyst that may extend by centric expansion, or more commonly in a pericentric fashion, to form a crescentic hole that progresses to a horseshoe tear [6]. Complete avulsion of the cyst roof results in a fully detached operculum that is suspended on the posterior vitreous cortex in the prefoveal plane [6, 7, 10]. Opercula primarily comprise vitreous cortex and glial elements with a variable amount of foveal tissue that includes photoreceptor cells in 40% of cases [11]. The photoreceptor layer, which is no longer anchored by the Muller cell cone at the foveola, undergoes passive centrifugal retraction to form a full-thickness retinal dehiscence with centrifugal displacement of xanthophyll [9, 12]. The edge of the hole becomes progressively elevated and a cuff of subretinal fluid develops. In the event of vitreo-foveal separation during the development of the macular hole, the relief of traction may result in regression of a cyst, but spontaneous closure of an established full-thickness macular hole is relatively uncommon [13].

While the majority of age-related macular holes are idiopathic in etiology, full-thickness macular holes may also occur in association with high myopia, following posterior segment surgery such as scleral buckling and pneumatic retinopexy, and following ocular trauma. Traumatic macular holes typically result from blunt injury, but have also been reported following laser injury and lightning strike.

Summary for the Clinician

- Idiopathic full-thickness macular holes are caused by traction exerted by the posterior vitreous cortex on the neurosensory retina at the fovea. Disinsertion of its glial plug results in the formation of a foveal "cyst." Avulsion of the cyst roof results in a free operculum suspended on the posterior vitreous cortex. The neurosensory retina retracts centrifugally to form a full-thickness retinal dehiscence.

1.3 Clinical Staging

Macular hole formation typically evolves through a series of four major stages that were first described according to their biomicroscopic features by Gass (Fig. 1.1, Table 1.1) [5, 14]. Stage 1 ('impending') macular hole is loss of the normal

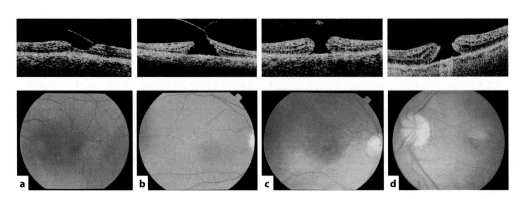

Fig. 1.1 Fundus photographs and OCT images of stage 1–4 macular holes. **a** Stage 1b lesion with a partial-thickness foveal defect. **b** Stage 2 full-thickness hole associated with persistent vitreo-foveal attachment. **c** Stage 3 full-thickness hole with separation of the vitreous from the macula and a fully detached operculum on the posterior hyaloid face. **d** Stage 4 full-thickness hole with complete posterior vitreous separation from the macula and optic disc

Table 1.1 Clinical features and natural history of idiopathic macular holes

	Stage 1	Stage 2	Stage 3	Stage 4
Symptoms	Asymptomatic, or mild metamorphopsia	Metamorphopsia and loss of central vision	Metamorphopsia and loss of central vision	Metamorphopsia and loss of central vision
Visual acuity	20/20–20/60	20/40–20/100	20/60–20/200	20/60–20/400
Biomicroscopy	Loss of foveal depression	Full-thickness retinal defect	Full-thickness retinal defect	Full-thickness retinal defect
	Yellow spot (1a) or yellow ring (1b)	Typically ≤200 µm in diameter	Typically 250–400 µm in diameter	Typically ≥450 µm in diameter
			Operculum may be evident	Operculum may be evident
	Posterior vitreous attached to fovea and optic disc	Posterior vitreous attached to fovea and optic disc	Posterior vitreous typically detached from fovea, but attached to optic disc	Posterior vitreous detached from both fovea and optic disc
Natural history	50% regress	15–21% regress	5% regress	
	40% progress	75% progress	30% progress	20% enlarge
	10% stabilize			

foveal depression, associated with the development of a yellow spot (stage 1a) or ring (stage 1b) in the centre of the fovea, changes that reflect the intraretinal schisis that progresses into an intraretinal cyst. A foveal dehiscence may be masked on biomicroscopy (stage 1-b, occult hole) by semi-opaque contracted prefoveolar vitreous cortex bridging the yellow ring. Stage 2 is a small full-thickness hole (≤200 µm), typically with a pericentric configuration, associated with persistent vitreo-foveal attachment. Stage 3 is a larger full-thickness hole (250–400 µm) with a rim of elevated retina and separation of the posterior hyaloid from the macula. A fully detached operculum on the posterior hyaloid may be evident on biomicroscopy. Stage 4 is a full-thickness hole (≥450 µm) with complete posterior vitreous separation from the optic disc, typically demonstrated by the presence of a Weiss ring.

1.4 Natural History

The natural history of macular holes is typically to progress in size and clinical stage, with deterioration in visual acuity that generally stabilizes at the 6/60 to 3/60 level, redistribution of yellow nodular opacities at the level of the retinal pigment epithelium, and the development of retinal pigment epithelial atrophy surrounding the macular hole, resulting in a 'bull's-eye' macular appearance.

An estimated 40% of stage 1 (impending) macular holes progress to full-thickness holes [15], but up to 50% resolve spontaneously [15, 16]. Stage 2 macular holes typically enlarge, with progression to stage 3 in at least 75% of cases [10, 16, 17] and spontaneous closure has been reported in no more than 15–21% [10, 13, 16]. Stage 3 holes progress to stage 4 in approximately 30% of cases over 3 years [16]. Full-thickness holes tend to enlarge modestly; by 25% during the first 12 months and by 29% at 24 months,

1

associated with a deterioration in mean visual acuity from 6/36 to 6/60. Spontaneous closure of stage 3 and stage 4 holes is rare, occurring in no more than 6% of cases [13].

While macular holes frequently stabilize at stage 3, they may resolve spontaneously with associated improvement in visual acuity at any stage during the course of their progression (Table 1.1). Spontaneous regression occurs in association with vitreo-foveal separation and is more likely during the early stages than during the later stages of macular hole evolution; it has been suggested that holes relieved of traction at an early stage may be more amenable to glial repair [13]. Spontaneous resolution of small full-thickness macular holes following trauma in young patients is not uncommon and can be associated with good visual recovery.

1.5 Risk of Full-Thickness Macular Hole in the Fellow Eye

The majority of full-thickness macular holes are unilateral. Since many affected individuals have normal visual acuity in their fellow eye at the time of presentation, the risk of macular hole development in the fellow eye is an important consideration in clinical management. While a stage 1 macular hole is associated with an estimated 40–50% risk of progression to a full-thickness hole, the presence of a complete posterior vitreous detachment, as indicated by a Weiss ring, is associated with a risk of progression of less than 1%. In normal fellow eyes without a Weiss ring the incidence of macular holes has been estimated as 7.5% at 18 months and 15.6% at 5 years after presentation [18]. In clinically normal fellow eyes, abnormalities in focal electroretinography and in color contrast sensitivity [18] suggest that subclinical foveal dysfunction appears to be predictive of an increased risk of macular hole development.

Summary for the Clinician

- Spontaneous regression of full-thickness macular holes, particularly stage 3 and stage 4, is uncommon.
- The risk of macular hole development in the fellow eye, in the absence of a Weiss ring, is 16% during the 5 years following presentation.

1.6 Symptoms and Signs

Many patients who have stage 1 macular holes and some with stage 2 holes are asymptomatic and are identified only on routine eye examination, particularly in cases where the fellow eye has normal acuity. Typical presenting features are progressive blurring of central vision and metamorphopsia, classically with micropsia and pin-cushion distortion, and occasionally a pericentral positive scotoma. Visual acuity may be relatively well preserved in stage 1 holes (6/6–6/24), but deteriorates with progression to stage 2 (6/12–6/36), and further to stage III (6/18–6/60) [5, 17]. The diagnosis of full-thickness macular holes and the stage of progression is generally established on the basis of the clinical history and biomicroscopic examination. The features of a full-thickness macular hole comprise a circular defect of the neurosensory retina, the edges of which are typically elevated by a cuff of subretinal fluid. Small yellow spots of xanthophyll pigment may be seen in the retinal pigment epithelium at the base of a full-thickness macular hole and an epiretinal membrane may be present overlying it. A small full-thickness foveal dehiscence may not be evident on biomicroscopy if it is obscured by semi-opaque contracted prefoveolar vitreous cortex (stage 1-b occult hole).

The differential diagnosis of stage 1 (impending) macular hole lesions includes cystoid macular edema, central serous retinopathy, vitelliform dystrophy, and pattern dystrophy lesions. The differential diagnosis of a full-thickness macular hole includes a pseudo-hole in an epiretinal membrane and a lamellar hole associated with arrested macular hole development or cystoid macular edema.

In some instances, differentiating full-thickness macular holes from pseudoholes on the basis of their clinical features alone can be difficult. Subjective distortion as described on Amsler grid testing is a sensitive sign, but has poor specificity for macular hole lesions [19]. Fundus contact lens examination offers an optimal view for biomicroscopy and the Watzke-Allen slit beam test can be a valuable sign if the diagnosis is uncertain. In the Watzke-Allen test a narrow vertical slit beam is projected across the fovea. The diagnosis of full-thickness macular hole is supported if the slit beam is perceived by the patient to be discontinuous (Watzke-Allen positive). This perception of discontinuity is believed to reflect the area of detached neuro-sensory retina as opposed to the centrifugal distraction of foveal photoreceptors or loss of photoreceptor elements. Patients who have small full-thickness holes, lamellar holes or epiretinal membranes may perceive the slit beam to be thinned, kinked or bowed. While the perception of discontinuity alone is a relatively insensitive sign, with careful interpretation the Watzke-Allen test may offer valuable information in the diagnosis of macular hole and may be predictive of visual prognosis postoperatively [12, 19]. The laser aiming beam test is performed in a similar way. The diagnosis of macular hole is supported if the patient is unable to perceive a 50-μm laser aiming beam projected within the lesion, but is able to do so when the beam is projected onto adjacent normal retina. The laser aiming beam is both sensitive and specific in differentiating clinically defined full-thickness macular holes from pseudoholes [19].

1.7 Fluorescein Angiography and Fundus Autofluorescence

Fundus fluorescein angiography can be a valuable technique in the management of macular holes when the diagnosis is in question. Stage 1 and stage 2 macular holes may be demonstrated by subtle focal hyperfluorescence at the fovea in the early phase, although this is not a reliable feature. The central hyperfluorescence is more marked in stage 3 and stage 4 holes and the cuff of subretinal fluid becomes apparent as a ring that may be hyperfluorescent or hypofluorescent [20].

Fundus autofluorescence imaging offers an alternative non-invasive and sensitive technique to aid the diagnosis and staging of macular holes [20]. Autofluorescence imaging of macular holes typically demonstrates bright fluorescence at the fovea similar to that demonstrated by fluorescein angiography, whereas macular pseudoholes demonstrate normal autofluorescence. The attached operculum in stage 2 macular holes and the pre-retinal operculum in stage 3 macular holes may cause focal masking of the background autofluorescence, a feature not evident on fluorescein angiography (Fig. 1.2). The cuff of neurosensory retinal detachment surrounding the macular hole demonstrates reduced autofluorescence.

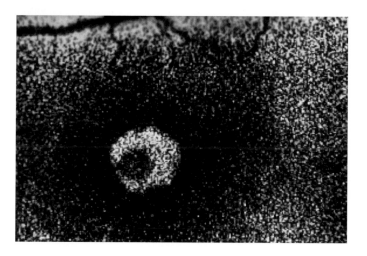

Fig. 1.2 Autofluorescence fundus image of a stage 3 macular hole. The central ring of hyperfluorescence corresponds to the full thickness neurosensory retinal defect. This is partly obscured by an overlying operculum

1.8 Optical Coherence Tomography

Optical coherence tomography (OCT) is a relatively novel non-invasive, non-contact imaging technique capable of producing cross-sectional images of ocular tissue in vivo of high longitudinal resolution (10 µm). OCT has not only yielded important insights into the pathogenesis of macular hole development and the mechanism of surgical repair, but also offers a valuable technique in clinical management. OCT is useful in the diagnosis of full-thickness macular holes, especially where there is uncertainty on biomicroscopy, and is able to distinguish full-thickness macular holes from partial thickness holes, macular pseudoholes, and cysts. OCT is also useful for defining the stage of macular hole development and providing a quantitative measure of hole size and associated macular edema. OCT has been used to evaluate the vitreoretinal interface in the fellow eyes of individuals with macular holes and enables the detection of subtle separations of the posterior hyaloid from the retina that are not evident clinically [21]. The configuration of macular holes on OCT can be predictive of postoperative visual outcome [7, 22, 23].

Ultrahigh-resolution OCT offers enhanced visualization of retinal architecture providing additional information on the morphology of macular disease and promises to improve the understanding of disease progression and its management [24].

Summary for the Clinician

■ The diagnosis and staging of macular holes is normally made on the basis of biomicroscopic features alone.

■ In instances where the diagnosis is in doubt, the Watzke-Allen slit beam test, the laser aiming beam test, fluorescein angiography or autofluorescence funduscopy may offer valuable additional information. Optical coherence tomography is particularly well suited to imaging of the retinal defect and the vitreoretinal interface.

1.9 Surgical Management of Macular Holes

The rationale for the surgical management of idiopathic macular holes, originally described by Kelly and Wendel in 1991 [25], is to relieve vitreo-foveal traction and to flatten and re-appose the macular hole edges by intraocular tamponade. This is achieved by three-port pars plana vitrectomy with meticulous removal of posterior cortical vitreous and of any epiretinal membranes at the macula. A peripheral vitrectomy is completed and the retinal periphery inspected for iatrogenic retinal breaks. An air-fluid exchange is performed and the intraocular air is usually exchanged for long-acting gas or silicone oil tamponade. Modifications of the original technique include peeling of the inner limiting membrane with or without local application of an adjuvant in an effort to promote healing by glial repair. Patients may be advised to posture in a face-down position for up to 14 days postoperatively.

The Vitrectomy for Prevention of Macular Hole (VPMH) study investigated the effect of surgery on reducing the risk of progression from stage 1 (impending) macular holes to full-thickness macular defects. This trial suggested that any benefit of vitrectomy in preventing progression to full-thickness macular holes is likely to be minimal and unlikely to outweigh the risk of surgical complications [15]. It was proposed that stage 1 holes should be observed by careful follow-up since only a minority of patients are likely to progress to full-thickness macular holes within a year. However, good anatomical and visual outcomes have been obtained in eyes with stage I holes and worsening vision, and in eyes with acute progression to full-thickness holes [26].

In eyes with full-thickness macular holes, vitrectomy with intraocular gas tamponade significantly improves the rate of both anatomical closure and visual function. Outcomes are particularly favorable for stage 2 holes and holes of less than 6 months' duration. In their original series, Kelly and Wendel reported an anatomical closure rate of 58%, and visual improvement in 73% of eyes in which holes were closed [25, 27]. Two large randomized controlled trials have since been conducted to determine the effect of vitrectomy and intraocular gas tamponade on the anatomical and visual outcomes. The Vitrectomy for Macular Hole Study (VMHS) was a multicenter trial that included 171 eyes followed for 12 months postoperatively [28, 29] and the Moorfields Macular Hole Study (MMHS) was a single surgeon trial that followed 185 eyes over 2 years [13]. In the MMHS the overall anatomic closure rate for stage 2, 3, and 4 macular holes was 81% at 24 months following surgery compared with 11% in the observation group, and surgery was associated with a significant reduction in macular hole dimensions [13]. Operated eyes improved in median Snellen acuity from 6/36 to 6/18, compared with a deterioration from 6/36 to 6/60 in the observation group. Median near acuity improved even more dramatically in the operated group from N10 to N5, compared with a deterioration from N10 to N14 over 24 months in the observation group. The number of eyes with Snellen acuity of 6/12 or better increased from 0% at baseline to 44% at 24 months in the operated group in contrast to the number in the observation group, which increased from 0% at baseline to 7% over the same period.

The VMHS demonstrated a clear benefit of surgical management in reducing the rate of progression of stage 2 to stage 3 or 4 macular holes. After 12 months' follow-up of 42 eyes, only 20% of the stage 2 macular holes randomized to vitrectomy progressed to stage 3 or 4 holes, compared with 71% of eyes in the observation group ($p=0.006$) [28]. While this study did not demonstrate a statistically significant effect on ETDRS visual acuity at 6 or 12 months, it was not statistically powered to detect modest differences and the study design precluded surgery for cataract that may have masked an improvement in potential visual acuity in eyes randomized to surgery. Indeed, operated eyes in this study did perform significantly better than un-operated eyes at word reading and on potential acuity meter testing, a measure less influenced by cataract development than ETDRS acuity. Since progression of macular holes from stage 2 is usually associated with deterioration in visual acuity, the clear benefit of surgery on anatomical progression demonstrated by this study is supportive of surgery for stage 2 holes. In the MMHS, 96% of treated stage 2 holes were closed at 24 months compared with 21% in the observation group that closed spontaneously

($p<0.001$). Surgery was associated with a mean difference of 2 Snellen lines of acuity [13].

Both the VMHS and the MMHS demonstrated a clear benefit of surgical management of stage 3 and stage 4 macular holes on the rate of anatomical closure and on final visual acuity. In the VMHS, after 6 months' follow-up of 129 eyes with stage 3 and stage 4 macular holes, anatomical closure was achieved in 69% of eyes randomized to surgery compared with only 4% of eyes randomized to observation alone ($p<0.001$). The surgically treated eyes had significantly better visual acuity at 6 months as measured ETDRS visual acuity (mean acuity was 20/115 in operated eyes vs. 20/166 in observed eyes, $p<0.01$) and higher word reading scores [29]. In the MMHS, anatomical closure was achieved in 77% of eyes with stage 3 and 4 holes randomized to surgery, compared with only 6% of eyes in the observation group ($p<0.001$), associated with a mean difference of 2 Snellen lines of acuity between the treatment groups [13]. The surgical techniques and results have improved since these two trials began and many case series now report primary anatomical closure following conventional surgery in approximately 80–90% of eyes with full-thickness macular holes [30–33].

Summary for the Clinician

- Evidence does not support the value of the surgical management of stage 1 (impending) macular holes.
- Vitrectomy and intraocular gas tamponade reduces the rate of macular hole progression and results in high rates of hole closure and visual improvement in eyes with full-thickness macular holes.

1.10 Technique for Conventional Macular Hole Surgery

- A three port pars plana core vitrectomy is performed.
- A complete posterior vitreous detachment is induced; the posterior hyaloid face at the optic disc is elevated by active aspiration using the

vitreous cutter or passively using a flute needle. Separation of the hyaloid from the retina is evident from the appearance of a Weiss ring and by an advancing wave-like demarcation line between attached and detached posterior hyaloid.

- Posterior cortical vitreous and any epiretinal membranes are meticulously removed using a pick and membrane forceps.
- A peripheral vitrectomy is completed and the retinal periphery is searched for iatrogenic breaks.
- An air–fluid exchange is performed and usually a long-acting gas is infused.
- Patients may be advised to posture face-down for up to 14 days postoperatively.

1.11 Tamponade Agents and Postoperative Posturing

Intraocular tamponade following vitrectomy for macular holes is believed to facilitate re-apposition of the rim of a detached neurosensory retina and to provide an interface with the vitreous fluid component that serves as a template for glial migration across the macular hole.

Consistently favorable anatomic and visual outcomes can be achieved by long-acting gas tamponade with strict face-down posturing as originally advocated [25]. In a comparative study of 52 eyes, use of 16% perfluoropropane gas resulted in anatomical closure in 97% and improvement in visual acuity by a mean of 3.1 lines, whereas use of air resulted in closure in only 53.3% and improved mean acuity by only 1.3 lines [34]. In another comparative series of 149 eyes, tamponade by 16% perfluoropropane and face-down posturing for 2 weeks resulted in an anatomical closure rate of 94%, compared with 65% following tamponade by lower concentrations of perfluoropropane and shorter durations of posturing; visual outcomes paralleled the rates of macular hole closure [35].

Prolonged face-down posturing is a task that presents a formidable challenge for many patients, and for some may be an unrealistic expectation. A number of studies have suggested that the use of shorter acting gases or shorter durations of face-down posturing can result in ana-

tomical and visual outcomes comparable to those of longer tamponade with a more rapid recovery of visual acuity postoperatively. In a nonrandomized comparative trial of 62 eyes, tamponade by 23% sulfahexafluoride and face-down posturing for 6 days resulted in anatomical closure in 93.5%, compared with 96.7% following tamponade by 16% perfluorodecaline and face-down posturing for 2–4 weeks. The final visual outcome was similar in both groups [36]. In a series of 58 eyes, macular hole surgery involving ILM peel, intraocular air tamponade, and face-down posturing for only 4 days resulted in a primary anatomical closure of 91% and final closure rate of 95% [37].

Good anatomic and visual outcomes have been reported following gas tamponade with no posturing at all when care is taken to ensure a complete intraocular gas fill. Combined cataract and vitrectomy surgery may facilitate optimal gas tamponade leading to good outcomes with no face-down posturing. In a series of 31 eyes, combined surgery with tamponade by 15% perfluoropropane, but no posturing resulted in primary anatomic closure in 79% and final closure in 85%. Forty-eight percent of eyes attained visual acuity of 20/50 [38]. In another series that included 20 eyes, combined surgery with tamponade by 20% C_2F_6, but no face-down posturing, resulted in anatomical closure in 90% and improvement in visual acuity by at least 0.3 logMAR units in 95% [39].

An alternative proposed for patients who are unable to perform prolonged face-down posturing is the use of silicone oil tamponade [40]. Macular hole surgery with the use of silicone oil and no posturing (except to avoid the face-up position) results in primary anatomic closure rates of 80–97% [40–42]. The rate of primary failure of hole closure may be reduced by ensuring an optimal oil fill [40]. The effect of silicone oil tamponade on visual outcome following macular hole surgery, however, is not clear. In one nonrandomized comparative trial of 54 eyes, visual outcome following silicone-oil tamponade was significantly better than following the use of short-acting gas; 74% of eyes achieved visual acuity of 6/12 or better following oil versus 47% following sulfahexafluoride [42]. Other reports have suggested that the use of silicone oil may be associated with a poorer visual outcome. In a series of 10 patients unable to perform prolonged face-down posturing, macular hole surgery using silicone oil tamponade resulted in an anatomical closure rate of 80%, but an improvement in visual acuity in only 38% of these eyes even after cataract surgery [41]. While this finding may reflect longer durations of macular holes in this selected group of patients, the possibility that silicone oil might have a toxic effect on the exposed outer retina at the macula suggests that its early removal may be advisable in this situation.

Summary for the Clinician

- Excellent outcomes can be achieved by long-acting intraocular gas tamponade with 10–14 days of face-down posturing.
- The use of shorter-acting gases and shorter durations of face-down posturing may also result in good anatomical and visual outcomes.
- For patients unable to perform face-down posturing, a complete fill of long-acting gas or silicone oil tamponade may be considered.

1.12 Biological Adjuncts to Macular Hole Surgery

The application of biological adjuncts to the macula during vitrectomy has been advocated with the aim of improving anatomical and functional outcomes by promoting glial repair of the hole after surgery. Biological adjuncts used in macular hole surgery have included transforming growth factor-beta 2 (TGF-β_2), autologous platelet concentrate (APC), autologous serum, and thrombin and fibrin mixtures.

In a randomized controlled trial including 90 patients, anatomical closure of full-thickness macular holes was achieved in 91% of eyes following local application of bovine TGF-β_2 compared with 53% in the placebo group. The visual results of this study were not reported [43]. While a small prospective randomized trial of different

doses of TGF-β_2 suggested a beneficial effect on visual outcome [44], studies of nonbovine (recombinant) TGF-β_2 demonstrated no significant benefit to vision. In a randomized controlled trial including 130 eyes, application of recombinant TGF-β resulted in anatomical closure in 78% of eyes compared with 61% in the placebo group ($p=0.08$), but there was no statistically significant difference in visual acuity between the groups [45].

Although the adjunctive use of APC in macular hole surgery results in a significantly higher rate of anatomical hole closure, no significant effect on functional outcome has been demonstrated. In a randomized controlled trial of surgery in 110 eyes the adjunctive use of APC resulted in 98% primary closure versus 82% in the control group ($p=0.009$), but visual acuity was not significantly different between the two groups [46] and subsequent study suggested relatively high rates of the late re-opening of macular holes.

The use of autologous serum is associated with no improvement in anatomical outcome [47]. In the MMHS, a randomized controlled trial of 185 eyes that addressed the effect of serum in addition to conventional surgery, the adjunctive use of autologous serum resulted in an anatomic closure rate that was only marginally higher than that of the control group at 24 months (83.1 vs. 78.0% respectively) with no significant differences in visual outcome [13].

In summary, while the intraoperative application of certain adjunctive biological agents may improve the rate of anatomical hole closure, none have been shown to result in a significant improvement in visual outcome.

Summary for the Clinician

- The application of biological adjunctive agents to the macula during vitrectomy has been advocated to promote glial repair of the hole after surgery.
- Certain adjunctive agents may improve the rate of hole closure, but there is no evidence that they improve visual outcomes.

1.13 Technique for Intraoperative Application of Biological Adjuncts

- Pars plana vitrectomy with dissection of posterior cortical vitreous and fluid–air exchange is performed.
- Up to 0.5 ml of the adjunctive agent is applied directly to the macular area and left for up to 10 min.
- The adjunct is then removed by passive aspiration using a cannula.
- Air–gas exchange is then performed.

1.14 Inner Limiting Membrane Peeling

Peeling of the inner limiting membrane (ILM) from the macula is a technique advocated in an attempt to further improve anatomical and visual outcomes of surgery for macular holes. The rationale for peeling the ILM is to relieve tangential traction from the edges of the hole and to promote closure by stimulation of wound healing. Peeling the ILM ensures thorough removal of any tangential tractional components implicated in the development of macular holes. The removal of a potential scaffold for re-proliferation of myofibroblasts may reduce the possibility of late re-opening of surgically closed holes. Furthermore, peeling of the ILM is also believed to stimulate wound healing at the macula, possibly by inducing local expression of undefined growth factors that promote glial repair.

There have been no randomized controlled trials to investigate the effect of ILM peeling on the outcome of macular hole surgery. The evidence currently available tends to support a benefit in terms of anatomical outcome, but the effect on visual function is less well established. A number of nonrandomized comparative series suggest that ILM peeling results in a higher rate of hole closure and that this is associated with improved visual outcomes. In one study of 160 eyes ILM peeling was associated with 100% hole closure rate and no re-openings, compared with 82% closure with 25% re-openings in the non-ILM peeled group [33]. In another comparative study of 39 eyes ILM peeling resulted in 90%

hole closure and improvement of visual acuity by 2 lines or more in 62%, compared with 50% closure and 44% improvement in acuity without ILM peeling [48]. In another study ILM peeling resulted in anatomical closure in 97.7% of 44 eyes versus 77.3% of 97 eyes without ILM peeling [49]. Visual acuity after surgery was 6/15 or better in 70.4% of eyes versus 56.7% of eyes, and increased by 2 or more lines in 77.3% eyes compared with 64.9% eyes respectively; the use of ILM peeling was associated with a greater than 2-fold increased probability of developing 6/15 vision or better [49]. Other studies, however, have not demonstrated any advantages of ILM peeling. In one nonrandomized comparative series of 107 eyes, an overall closure rate of 89% was achieved with visual acuity improving by 2 lines or more in 85% of eyes; ILM peeling was associated with no statistically significant difference in closure rate or visual outcome [32].

While ILM peeling may improve the rate of anatomical closure, evidence suggests that it can result in an adverse effect on visual function. In one series, ILM peeling resulted in anatomical closure in 100% of 29 eyes compared with 85.1% of 27 eyes without ILM peeling. In eyes with holes that were successfully closed, however, visual improvement of 3 or more lines at 3 months was achieved in only 44.8% following ILM peeling versus 79.2% of 24 eyes without ILM peeling ($p=0.01$) [50]. In another series that included 193 eyes with macular holes, ILM peeling was attempted in all cases. Although anatomical closure achieved after complete ILM peeling was associated with improved visual outcomes, the rate of anatomic closure was inversely correlated with the extent of ILM peeling actually achieved. It was suggested that excessive unsuccessful attempts at ILM peeling might enhance anatomic success (possibly through enhanced promotion of glial healing) at the expense of poorer visual outcome, presumably resulting from damage to inner retinal elements [51]. Small paracentral scotomata have been observed on microperimetry in more than 50% of eyes in which ILM peeling has been attempted, possibly due to direct trauma resulting in small defects in the nerve fiber layer. The scotomata may be multiple, but are generally asymptomatic, nonprogressive and not associated with any significant effect on visual acuity [52]. ILM peeling can also result in a punctate chorio-retinopathy [53] and in delayed recovery of the macular focal electroretinogram b-wave, suggesting an alteration of retinal physiology in the macular region [54].

Inner limiting membrane peeling appears to improve the rate of anatomical closure, but its effect on visual outcome is less predictable and excessive unsuccessful attempts to peel the ILM are associated with poor visual outcome. While ILM peeling may be performed for full-thickness macular holes of any stage, it is more commonly reserved for stage 3 or 4 holes, long-standing holes, those that have failed to close, or those that have re-opened following conventional surgery.

Summary for the Clinician

- The rationale for peeling the ILM is to promote macular hole closure by relief of tangential traction and stimulation of wound healing.
- Peeling of the ILM is associated with higher rates of anatomical closure.
- Persistent unsuccessful attempts to peel the ILM may be associated with poor visual outcome despite anatomical closure.

1.15 Technique for Inner Limiting Membrane Peeling

- Use a pick or micro-vitreoretinal blade to create an opening in the internal limiting membrane in the macular area at a location outside the maculo-papillary bundle, ideally along the temporal horizontal nerve fiber raphe.
- Use fine intraocular membrane forceps to grasp and elevate the ILM.
- The ILM can be difficult to visualizes, but is identified by its characteristic light reflex.
- Peel the ILM in a circular motion, in a manner similar to the technique of capsulorhexis in cataract surgery.
- Peel the ILM toward (not away from) the macular hole in order to avoid inadvertent enlargement of the hole.

- A characteristically pale dull reflex identifies areas of the macula successfully denuded of ILM.
- The ILM is usually removed from an area of the macular extending toward the vascular arcades.

1.16 Vital Staining to Facilitate Inner Limiting Membrane Peeling

Inner limiting membrane peeling is a technically challenging maneuver, in part because of the difficulty in distinguishing the ILM from the posterior vitreous cortex and the nerve fiber layer of the retina with confidence. As previously described, inadvertent injury to the nerve fiber layer can cause paracentral scotomata [52], and unsuccessful ILM peeling can result in poor visual outcome [51]. In order to achieve reproducible, complete, atraumatic ILM peeling the use of a vital dye has been advocated to facilitate its clear identification.

1.17 Indocyanine Green

Indocyanine green (ICG) dye selectively stains the ILM. The improved contrast between the green ICG-stained ILM and the unstained underlying retina facilitates initiation of the peel and enables precise monitoring of its extent. Furthermore, the application of ICG is believed to create a cleavage plane that facilitates removal of the ILM.

Indocyanine green-assisted ILM peeling is associated with high rates of macular hole closure. In a nonrandomized comparative trial of 68 eyes, macular hole surgery with ICG-assisted ILM peel (5 mg/ml) resulted in 91.2% primary closure rate and 82% improvement in visual acuity above baseline, versus 73.5% primary closure rate and 53% improvement in vision following ILM peeling without ICG ($p=0.056$) [55]. In other series surgery with ICG-assisted ILM peeling resulted in anatomic closure in 88–97% of cases [56–58].

Although at least one large series has identified no significant adverse effects of 0.5% IGC-assisted ILM peeling even in the long term [59], others suggest that the use of ICG can be associated with poorer visual outcomes despite high rates of anatomical closure. In a nonrandomized comparative study of 79 eyes, ICG-assisted ILM peeling resulted in anatomical closure in 97.1% versus 97.7% without ICG. Postoperative visual acuity, however, was 20/50 or better in only 51.4% of eyes following ICG use versus 70.4% without ICG [49]. Several series have reported high rates of anatomical closure with no significant improvement in visual acuity [60–63]. Moreover, the use of ICG has been associated with the development of irreversible peripheral nasal–visual field defects, consistent with retinal nerve fiber damage involving predominantly the temporal retina [60, 61, 63].

The reason for poor visual acuity and unexpected visual field defects reported in association with the use of ICG is not well understood.

Mechanical, toxic or phototoxic mechanisms may be involved. Analysis of ILM peeled after ICG-staining has demonstrated adherence of additional retinal elements including remnants of Müller cell footplates, neuronal cells, and ganglion cells suggesting that ICG may alter the cleavage plane to involve the innermost retinal layers [64]. A number of studies have suggested that ICG may be toxic to exposed retinal pigment epithelium at the base of the macular hole. ICG-related retinal hyperfluorescence persists for up to 9 months following intravitreal application and unusual retinal pigment epithelial changes in the area of the macular hole have been noted postoperatively in a high proportion of eyes [62]. Application of ICG induces degeneration of outer retinal cells and an adverse effect on retinal function in experimental models [65]. ICG can induce phototoxic injury in retinal pigment epithelial cells in vitro [66] and evidence suggests that the spectral absorption properties of ICG may result in a phototoxic effect at the vitreoretinal interface [67].

The inconsistent effects of ICG on visual outcome reported in the literature may reflect the differences in concentrations of dye and durations of exposure [68]. Further investigations are required to determine whether a safe technique for the ICG staining of the ILM in macular hole surgery can be defined. In the meantime low concentrations of ICG and brief duration of applica-

tion are preferred. The application of perfluorocarbon liquid, viscoelastic or whole blood to the macular hole prior to ICG staining has been advocated to protect the exposed foveal RPE from possible toxic effects [69]. In view of a possible phototoxic effect, the intensity and duration of endoillumination should also be minimized.

1.18   Trypan Blue

Trypan blue dye offers an alternative to ICG for ILM staining (Fig. 1.3). Trypan blue effectively stains the ILM facilitating its dissection resulting in the anatomical closure of macular holes in 94–100% of eyes [70–72]. No significant adverse effect related to the use of trypan blue has been reported up to 1 year postoperatively, but further studies are required to investigate its long-term safety.

Summary for the Clinician

- Indocyanine green and trypan blue dyes facilitate identification and dissection of the ILM.
- The use of ICG results in high rates of macular hole closure, but can be associated with poor visual outcomes.
- Indocyanine green should be used with caution until a safe technique for its application is established.
- Trypan blue dye is a valuable alternative that appears to have a good safety profile in initial studies.

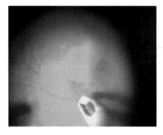

Fig. 1.3 Intraoperative photograph showing peeling of the inner limiting membrane stained by trypan blue

1.19 Technique for Inner Limiting Membrane Staining

- Indocyanine green dye is reconstituted to attain a final concentration of 0.125–0.5%.
- Trypan blue is used at a concentration of 0.06%.
- Following pars plana vitrectomy, up to 0.5 ml of dye is instilled under fluid or air directly into the posterior vitreous cavity over the macula and the infusion is temporarily stopped.
- Dye is left in the vitreous cavity for a period of 10 s to 5 min before removal by aspiration.
- Peeling of the ILM is then performed under fluid as described above.

1.20 Complications of Macular Hole Surgery

Peeling of the posterior vitreous cortex from the retinal surface can result in iatrogenic retinal tears. In the MMHS, retinal tears occurred in 3.2% of eyes and were effectively treated intraoperatively by retinopexy [13]. Retinal detachments occurred in 5.6% of eyes in the MMHS and in 11% of eyes in the VMHS [73]. Retinal detachments generally occur within the first 6–8 weeks postoperatively and have a high success rate of anatomic re-attachment following further surgery [13]. Although retinal detachment does not preclude improved final visual acuity, involvement of the macula and the development of proliferative vitreo-retinopathy indicate poorer prognosis [13].

Transient elevation of intraocular pressure is very common postoperatively and intraocular pressures of greater than 30 mmHg have been reported in over 50% of patients following tamponade by 14% perfluoropropane gas [74]. Transient elevation of intraocular pressure can generally be controlled by appropriate topical medication.

Postoperative peripheral visual field defects, consistent with damage to the retinal nerve fiber layer, have been described in up to 17% of cases [13, 75]. These visual field defects are believed to result from damage to the nerve fiber layer by the infusion of dry air under high pressure; the incidence of the field defects is dependent on the air pressure and its position is consistently lo-

cated contralateral to the site of the infusion cannula, whether placed temporally or nasally [76]. The development of field defects can be almost eliminated by limiting the air infusion pressure to 30 mmHg [77].

The development of cataract is almost inevitable following macular hole surgery. Lens opacity has been reported in 46% of eyes at 3 months postoperatively [75], and in greater than 80% by 2 years [33]. Since the development of cataract is predictable, combined cataract and vitrectomy surgery for macular hole has been advocated in order to obviate the requirement for subsequent cataract surgery [78]. Combined surgery has the added advantages afforded by excellent visibility of the retina per-operatively and a large fill of intraocular gas for optimal tamponade.

Alterations in the retinal pigment epithelium have been reported in as many as 33% of eyes following macular hole surgery [73]. Retinal pigment epitheliopathy, which has been attributed to surgical trauma or phototoxicity, may limit visual outcome and predispose to the development of choroidal neovascularization. Rarer complications of macular hole surgery include cystoid macular edema (1%) and postoperative endophthalmitis (1%) [73].

1.21 Prognosis Following Macular Hole Surgery

Visual recovery following surgical closure of macular holes may be gradual. Although substantial improvement in visual acuity occurs soon after cataract extraction, further improvement may be observed for up to 2 years [79]. Visual recovery is inversely correlated with vision in the fellow eye, tending to be greater where vision in the fellow eye is subnormal [80]. Bilateral visual function improves in a significant proportion of patients after macular hole surgery, particularly where vision in the fellow eye is subnormal [30]. Successful closure improves stereoacuity [81] and has a beneficial effect on patients' subjective perception of visual function [82], but the effect of macular hole surgery on patients' quality of life has yet to be fully evaluated.

The outcome of macular hole surgery is dependent on the stage of the hole and the duration

1

of symptoms, but is not dependent on the age of the patient. Anatomic and visual outcomes are inversely correlated to the stage of the hole and are greatest following surgery for small stage 2 holes [13]. The closure rate in patients undergoing surgery within 1 year of onset is 94.0%, and in those waiting 1 year or more it is 47.4% [83]. Although the best functional results are obtained if surgery is performed within 6 months of the onset of symptoms, visual improvement may be achieved in patients who have been symptomatic for much longer [84, 85]. Surgery for macular holes secondary to trauma can result in closure rates comparable to those of idiopathic holes, but high myopia or the presence of a localized macular detachment are associated with a relatively poor prognosis.

Following failure of primary surgery to close macular holes, further surgery involving rigorous dissection of epiretinal membranes, with or without ILM peeling, and long-acting gas tamponade can result in anatomical closure and improvement in visual acuity [86]. Alternatively, in eyes with unclosed macular holes following vitrectomy with ILM peeling, additional gas injection during the early postoperative period can result in successful closure [87]. In the MMHS, eyes in which hole closure was achieved after a second procedure attained slightly poorer LogMAR and Snellen acuities than eyes in which closure had been achieved after a single procedure, but achieved similar near acuities [13].

Summary for the Clinician

- The outcome following macular hole surgery is dependent on the duration and stage of the hole.
- Surgery for large and long-standing macular holes can result in a significant improvement in visual function.
- Following primary failure of surgery, reoperation can result in anatomical closure and improved visual acuity.

References

1. Evans JR, Schwartz SD, McHugh JD, Thamby-Rajah Y, Hodgson SA, Wormald RP, et al. Systemic risk factors for idiopathic macular holes: a case-control study. Eye. 1998;12(Pt 2):256–259.
2. Kang HK, Chang AA, Beaumont PE. The macular hole: report of an Australian surgical series and meta-analysis of the literature. Clin Exp Ophthalmol. 2000;28(4):298–308.
3. Lewis ML, Cohen SM, Smiddy WE, Gass JD. Bilaterality of idiopathic macular holes. Graefes Arch Clin Exp Ophthalmol. 1996;234(4):241–215.
4. Ezra E. Idiopathic full thickness macular hole: natural history and pathogenesis. Br J Ophthalmol. 2001;85(1):102–108.
5. Gass JD. Idiopathic senile macular hole. Its early stages and pathogenesis. Arch Ophthalmol. 1988;106(5):629–639.
6. Gaudric A, Haouchine B, Massin P, Paques M, Blain P, Erginay A. Macular hole formation: new data provided by optical coherence tomography. Arch Ophthalmol. 1999;117(6):744–751.
7. Tanner V, Chauhan DS, Jackson TL, Williamson TH. Optical coherence tomography of the vitreoretinal interface in macular hole formation. Br J Ophthalmol. 2001;85(9):1092–1097.
8. Azzolini C, Patelli F, Brancato R. Correlation between optical coherence tomography data and biomicroscopic interpretation of idiopathic macular hole. Am J Ophthalmol. 2001;132(3):348–355.
9. Gass JD. Muller cell cone, an overlooked part of the anatomy of the fovea centralis: hypotheses concerning its role in the pathogenesis of macular hole and foveomacular retinoschisis. Arch Ophthalmol. 1999;117(6):821–823.
10. Kim JW, Freeman WR, el-Haig W, Maguire AM, Arevalo JF, Azen SP. Baseline characteristics, natural history, and risk factors to progression in eyes with stage 2 macular holes. Results from a prospective randomized clinical trial. Vitrectomy for Macular Hole Study Group. Ophthalmology. 1995;102(12):1818–1828; discussion 28–29.
11. Ezra E, Munro PM, Charteris DG, Aylward WG, Luthert PJ, Gregor ZJ. Macular hole opercula. Ultrastructural features and clinicopathological correlation. Arch Ophthalmol. 1997;115(11):1381–1387.

12. Tanner V, Williamson TH. Watzke-Allen slit beam test in macular holes confirmed by optical coherence tomography. Arch Ophthalmol. 2000;118(8):1059–1063.

13. Ezra E, Gregor ZJ. Surgery for idiopathic full-thickness macular hole: two-year results of a randomized clinical trial comparing natural history, vitrectomy, and vitrectomy plus autologous serum: Morfields Macular Hole Study Group Report no. 1. Arch Ophthalmol. 2004;122(2):224–236.

14. Gass JD. Reappraisal of biomicroscopic classification of stages of development of a macular hole. Am J Ophthalmol. 1995;119(6):752–759.

15. De Bustros S. Vitrectomy for prevention of macular holes. Results of a randomized multicenter clinical trial. Vitrectomy for Prevention of Macular Hole Study Group. Ophthalmology. 1994;101(6):1055–1059; discussion 60.

16. Hikichi T, Yoshida A, Akiba J, Trempe CL. Natural outcomes of stage 1, 2, 3, and 4 idiopathic macular holes. Br J Ophthalmol. 1995;79(6):517–520.

17. Johnson RN, Gass JD. Idiopathic macular holes. Observations, stages of formation, and implications for surgical intervention. Ophthalmology. 1988;95(7):917–924.

18. Ezra E, Wells JA, Gray RH, Kinsella FM, Orr GM, Grego J, et al. Incidence of idiopathic full-thickness macular holes in fellow eyes. A 5-year prospective natural history study. Ophthalmology. 1998;105(2):353–359.

19. Martinez J, Smiddy WE, Kim J, Gass JD. Differentiating macular holes from macular pseudoholes. Am J Ophthalmol. 1994;117(6):762–767.

20. Von Ruckmann A, Fitzke FW, Gregor ZJ. Fundus autofluorescence in patients with macular holes imaged with a laser scanning ophthalmoscope. Br J Ophthalmol. 1998;82(4):346–351.

21. Hee MR, Puliafito CA, Wong C, Duker JS, Reichel E, Schuman JS, et al. Optical coherence tomography of macular holes. Ophthalmology. 1995;102(5):748–756.

22. Apostolopoulos MN, Koutsandrea CN, Moschos MN, Alonistiotis DA, Papaspyrou AE, Mallias JA, et al. Evaluation of successful macular hole surgery by optical coherence tomography and multifocal electroretinography. Am J Ophthalmol. 2002;134(5):667–674.

23. Kusuhara S, Teraoka Escano MF, Fujii S, Nakanishi Y, Tamura Y, Nagai A, et al. Prediction of postoperative visual outcome based on hole configuration by optical coherence tomography in eyes with idiopathic macular holes. Am J Ophthalmol. 2004;138(5):709–716.

24. Ko TH, Fujimoto JG, Schuman JS, Paunescu LA, Kowalevicz AM, Hartl I, et al. Comparison of ultrahigh- and standard-resolution optical coherence tomography for imaging macular pathology. Ophthalmology. 2005;112(11):1922.

25. Kelly NE, Wendel RT. Vitreous surgery for idiopathic macular holes. Results of a pilot study. Arch Ophthalmol. 1991;109(5):654–659.

26. Kokame GT. Management options for early stages of acutely symptomatic macular holes. Am J Ophthalmol. 2002;133(2):276–278.

27. Wendel RT, Patel AC, Kelly NE, Salzano TC, Wells JW, Novack GD. Vitreous surgery for macular holes. Ophthalmology. 1993;100(11):1671–1676.

28. Kim JW, Freeman WR, Azen SP, el-Haig W, Klein DJ, Bailey IL. Prospective randomized trial of vitrectomy or observation for stage 2 macular holes. Vitrectomy for Macular Hole Study Group. Am J Ophthalmol. 1996;121(6):605–614.

29. Freeman WR, Azen SP, Kim JW, el-Haig W, Mishell DR III, Bailey I. Vitrectomy for the treatment of full-thickness stage 3 or 4 macular holes. Results of a multicentered randomized clinical trial. The Vitrectomy for Treatment of Macular Hole Study Group. Arch Ophthalmol. 1997;115(1):11–21.

30. Polk TD, Smiddy WE, Flynn HW Jr. Bilateral visual function after macular hole surgery. Ophthalmology. 1996;103(3):422–426.

31. Smiddy WE, Pimentel S, Williams GA. Macular hole surgery without using adjunctive additives. Ophthalmic Surg Lasers. 1997;28(9):713–717.

32. Margherio RR, Margherio AR, Williams GA, Chow DR, Banach MJ. Effect of perifoveal tissue dissection in the management of acute idiopathic full-thickness macular holes. Arch Ophthalmol. 2000;118(4):495–498.

33. Brooks HL Jr. Macular hole surgery with and without internal limiting membrane peeling. Ophthalmology. 2000;107(10):1939–1948; discussion 48–49.

34. Thompson JT, Glaser BM, Sjaarda RN, Murphy RP, Hanham A. Effects of intraocular bubble duration in the treatment of macular holes by vitrectomy and transforming growth factor-beta 2. Ophthalmology. 1994;101(7):1195–1200.

35. Thompson JT, Smiddy WE, Glaser BM, Sjaarda RN, Flynn HW Jr. Intraocular tamponade duration and success of macular hole surgery. Retina. 1996;16(5):373–382.

36. Mulhern MG, Cullinane A, Cleary PE. Visual and anatomical success with short-term macular tamponade and autologous platelet concentrate. Graefes Arch Clin Exp Ophthalmol. 2000;238(7):577–583.

37. Park DW, Sipperley JO, Sneed SR, Dugel PU, Jacobsen J. Macular hole surgery with internal-limiting membrane peeling and intravitreous air. Ophthalmology. 1999;106(7):1392–1397; discussion 1397–1398.

38. Tornambe PE, Poliner LS, Grote K. Macular hole surgery without face-down positioning. A pilot study. Retina. 1997;17(3):179–185.

39. Simcock PR, Scalia S. Phacovitrectomy without prone posture for full thickness macular holes. Br J Ophthalmol. 2001;85(11):1316–1319.

40. Goldbaum MH, McCuen BW, Hanneken AM, Burgess SK, Chen HH. Silicone oil tamponade to seal macular holes without position restrictions. Ophthalmology. 1998;105(11):2140–2147; discussion 2147–2148.

41. Karia N, Laidlaw A, West J, Ezra E, Gregor MZ. Macular hole surgery using silicone oil tamponade. Br J Ophthalmol. 2001;85(11):1320–1323.

42. Pertile G, Claes C. Silicone oil vs. gas for the treatment of full-thickness macular hole. Bull Soc Belge Ophtalmol. 1999;274:31–36.

43. Smiddy WE, Glaser BM, Thompson JT, Sjaarda RN, Flynn HW Jr, Hanham A, et al. Transforming growth factor-beta 2 significantly enhances the ability to flatten the rim of subretinal fluid surrounding macular holes. Preliminary anatomic results of a multicenter prospective randomized study. Retina. 1993;13(4):296–301.

44. Glaser BM, Michels RG, Kuppermann BD, Sjaarda RN, Pena RA. Transforming growth factor-beta 2 for the treatment of full-thickness macular holes. A prospective randomized study. Ophthalmology. 1992;99(7):1162–1172; discussion 73.

45. Thompson JT, Smiddy WE, Williams GA, Sjaarda RN, Flynn HW Jr, Margherio RR, et al. Comparison of recombinant transforming growth factor-beta-2 and placebo as an adjunctive agent for macular hole surgery. Ophthalmology. 1998;105(4):700–706.

46. Paques M, Chastang C, Mathis A, Sahel J, Massin P, Dosquet C, et al. Effect of autologous platelet concentrate in surgery for idiopathic macular hole: results of a multicenter, double-masked, randomized trial. Platelets in Macular Hole Surgery Group. Ophthalmology. 1999;106(5):932–938.

47. Banker AS, Freeman WR, Azen SP, Lai MY. A multicentered clinical study of serum as adjuvant therapy for surgical treatment of macular holes. Vitrectomy for Macular Hole Study Group. Arch Ophthalmol. 1999;117(11):1499–1502.

48. Foulquier S, Glacet-Bernard A, Sterkers M, Soubrane G, Coscas G. [Study of internal limiting membrane peeling in stage-3 and -4 idiopathic macular hole surgery]. J Fr Ophtalmol. 2002;25(10):1026–1031.

49. Sheidow TG, Blinder KJ, Holekamp N, Joseph D, Shah G, Grand MG, et al. Outcome results in macular hole surgery: an evaluation of internal limiting membrane peeling with and without indocyanine green. Ophthalmology. 2003;110(9):1697–1701.

50. Al-Abdulla NA, Thompson JT, Sjaarda RN. Results of macular hole surgery with and without epiretinal dissection or internal limiting membrane removal. Ophthalmology. 2004;111(1):142–149.

51. Smiddy WE, Feuer W, Cordahi G. Internal limiting membrane peeling in macular hole surgery. Ophthalmology. 2001;108(8):1471–1476; discussion 1477–1478.

52. Haritoglou C, Gass CA, Schaumberger M, Gandorfer A, Ulbig MW, Kampik A. Long-term follow-up after macular hole surgery with internal limiting membrane peeling. Am J Ophthalmol. 2002;134(5):661–666.

53. Karacorlu M, Karacorlu S, Ozdemir H. Iatrogenic punctate chorioretinopathy after internal limiting membrane peeling. Am J Ophthalmol. 2003;135(2):178–182.

54. Terasaki H, Miyake Y, Nomura R, Piao CH, Hori K, Niwa T, et al. Focal macular ERGs in eyes after removal of macular ILM during macular hole surgery. Invest Ophthalmol Vis Sci. 2001;42(1):229–234.

55. Lochhead J, Jones E, Chui D, Lake S, Karia N, Patel CK, et al. Outcome of ICG-assisted ILM peel in macular hole surgery. Eye. 2004;18(8):804–808.

56. Da Mata AP, Burk SE, Riemann CD, Rosa RH Jr, Snyder ME, Petersen MR, et al. Indocyanine green-assisted peeling of the retinal internal limiting membrane during vitrectomy surgery for macular hole repair. Ophthalmology. 2001;108(7):1187–1192.

57. Van De Moere A, Stalmans P. Anatomical and visual outcome of macular hole surgery with infracyanine green-assisted peeling of the internal limiting membrane, endodrainage, and silicone oil tamponade. Am J Ophthalmol. 2003;136(5):879–887.

58. Wolf S, Reichel MB, Wiedemann P, Schnurrbusch UE. Clinical findings in macular hole surgery with indocyanine green-assisted peeling of the internal limiting membrane. Graefes Arch Clin Exp Ophthalmol. 2003;241(7):589–592.

59. Da Mata AP, Burk SE, Foster RE, Riemann CD, Petersen MR, Nehemy MB, et al. Long-term follow-up of indocyanine green-assisted peeling of the retinal internal limiting membrane during vitrectomy surgery for idiopathic macular hole repair. Ophthalmology. 2004;111(12):2246–2253.

60. Haritoglou C, Gandorfer A, Gass CA, Schaumberger M, Ulbig MW, Kampik A. Indocyanine green-assisted peeling of the internal limiting membrane in macular hole surgery affects visual outcome: a clinicopathologic correlation. Am J Ophthalmol. 2002;134(6):836–841.

61. Gass CA, Haritoglou C, Schaumberger M, Kampik A. Functional outcome of macular hole surgery with and without indocyanine green-assisted peeling of the internal limiting membrane. Graefes Arch Clin Exp Ophthalmol. 2003;241(9):716–720.

62. Engelbrecht NE, Freeman J, Sternberg P Jr, Aaberg TM Sr, Aaberg TM Jr, Martin DF, et al. Retinal pigment epithelial changes after macular hole surgery with indocyanine green-assisted internal limiting membrane peeling. Am J Ophthalmol. 2002;133(1):89–94.

63. Ando F, Sasano K, Ohba N, Hirose H, Yasui O. Anatomic and visual outcomes after indocyanine green-assisted peeling of the retinal internal limiting membrane in idiopathic macular hole surgery. Am J Ophthalmol. 2004;137(4):609–614.

64. La Heij EC, Dieudonne SC, Mooy CM, Diederen RM, Liem AT, van Suylen RJ, et al. Immunohistochemical analysis of the internal limiting membrane peeled with infracyanine green. Am J Ophthalmol. 2005;140(6):1123–1125.

65. Lee JE, Yoon TJ, Oum BS, Lee JS, Choi HY. Toxicity of indocyanine green injected into the subretinal space: subretinal toxicity of indocyanine green. Retina. 2003;23(5):675–681.

66. Sippy BD, Engelbrecht NE, Hubbard GB, Moriarty SE, Jiang S, Aaberg TM Jr, et al. Indocyanine green effect on cultured human retinal pigment epithelial cells: implication for macular hole surgery. Am J Ophthalmol. 2001;132(3):433–435.

67. Gandorfer A, Haritoglou C, Kampik A. Retinal damage from indocyanine green in experimental macular surgery. Invest Ophthalmol Vis Sci. 2003;44(1):316–323.

68. Ando F, Sasano K, Suzuki F, Ohba N. Indocyanine green-assisted ILM peeling in macular hole surgery revisited. Am J Ophthalmol. 2004;138(5):886–887.

69. Lai CC, Wu WC, Chuang LH, Yeung L, Chen TL, Lin KK. Prevention of indocyanine green toxicity on retinal pigment epithelium with whole blood in stain-assisted macular hole surgery. Ophthalmology. 2005;112(8):1409–1414.

70. Li K, Wong D, Hiscott P, Stanga P, Groenewald C, McGalliard J. Trypan blue staining of internal limiting membrane and epiretinal membrane during vitrectomy: visual results and histopathological findings. Br J Ophthalmol. 2003;87(2):216–219.

71. Teba FA, Mohr A, Eckardt C, Wong D, Kusaka S, Joondeph BC, et al. Trypan blue staining in vitreoretinal surgery. Ophthalmology. 2003;110(12):2409–2412.

72. Perrier M, Sebag M. Trypan blue-assisted peeling of the internal limiting membrane during macular hole surgery. Am J Ophthalmol. 2003;135(6):903–905.

73. Banker AS, Freeman WR, Kim JW, Munguia D, Azen SP. Vision-threatening complications of surgery for full-thickness macular holes. Vitrectomy for Macular Hole Study Group. Ophthalmology. 1997;104(9):1442–1452; discussion 1452–1453.

74. Chen CJ. Glaucoma after macular hole surgery. Ophthalmology. 1998;105(1):94–99; discussion 99–100.

75. Pearce IA, Branley M, Groenewald C, McGalliard J, Wong D. Visual function and patient satisfaction after macular hole surgery. Eye. 1998;12(Pt 4):651–658.

76. Hirata A, Yonemura N, Hasumura T, Murata Y, Negi A. Effect of infusion air pressure on visual field defects after macular hole surgery. Am J Ophthalmol. 2000;130(5):611–616.

77. Gass CA, Haritoglou C, Messmer EM, Schaumberger M, Kampik A. Peripheral visual field defects after macular hole surgery: a complication with decreasing incidence. Br J Ophthalmol. 2001;85(5):549–551.

78. Simcock PR, Scalia S. Phaco-vitrectomy for full-thickness macular holes. Acta Ophthalmol Scand. 2000;78(6):684–686.

79. Leonard RE II, Smiddy WE, Flynn HW Jr, Feuer W. Long-term visual outcomes in patients with successful macular hole surgery. Ophthalmology. 1997;104(10):1648–1652.

80. Kadonosono K, Yabuki K, Nishide T, Uchio E, Marron JA. Measured visual acuity of fellow eyes as a prognostic factor in macular hole surgery. Am J Ophthalmol. 2003;135(4):493–498.

81. Mireskandari K, Garnham L, Sheard R, Ezra E, Gregor ZJ, Sloper JJ. A prospective study of the effect of a unilateral macular hole on sensory and motor binocular function and recovery following successful surgery. Br J Ophthalmol. 2004;88(10):1320–1324.

82. Tranos PG, Ghazi-Nouri SM, Rubin GS, Adams ZC, Charteris DG. Visual function and subjective perception of visual ability after macular hole surgery. Am J Ophthalmol. 2004;138(6):995–1002.

83. Jaycock PD, Bunce C, Xing W, Thomas D, Poon W, Gazzard G, et al. Outcomes of macular hole surgery: implications for surgical management and clinical governance. Eye. 2005;19(8):879–884.

84. Scott RA, Ezra E, West JF, Gregor ZJ. Visual and anatomical results of surgery for long standing macular holes. Br J Ophthalmol. 2000;84(2):150–153.

85. Stec LA, Ross RD, Williams GA, Trese MT, Margherio RR, Cox MS Jr. Vitrectomy for chronic macular holes. Retina. 2004;24(3):341–347.

86. Ezra E, Aylward WG, Gregor ZJ. Membranectomy and autologous serum for the retreatment of full-thickness macular holes. Arch Ophthalmol. 1997;115(10):1276–1280.

87. Imai M, Gotoh T, Iijima H. Additional intravitreal gas injection in the early postoperative period for an unclosed macular hole treated with internal limiting membrane peeling. Retina. 2005;25(2):158–161.

Chapter 2

Heavy Silicone Oil for Persistent Macular Holes

2

Stanislao Rizzo, Federica Genovesi-Ebert

Core Messages

- The current surgical treatment consists of pars plana vitrectomy, peeling of the internal limiting membrane (ILM) with intraocular tamponading using long-acting gas. This technique can achieve macular hole (MH) closure in over 90% of cases. Indeed, in some cases anatomical closure is not obtained (persistent MH) and visual improvement is poor.

- Many surgeons give up treatment after one or two attempts at surgery.

- Inner limiting membrane (ILM) peeling and autologous platelets concentrate application after the failure of the first attempt at surgery for MH increases the anatomic success rate from 82 to 96%.

- With heavier than water silicone oil (HSO) for the treatment of persistent macular holes, anatomic closure was achieved in all patients.

- Optical coherence tomography (OCT) images showed that HSO, due to its specific gravity, achieved effective endotamponading of the foveal region in the upright position, allowing good anatomic and functional recovery.

- The exclusion of the fluid from the surface of the MH may avoid concentration of substance in the foveal region and is critical in favoring the MH seal and preventing epiretinal re-proliferation.

2.1. Introduction

2.1.1 Basics

Successful surgery for idiopathic macular holes (MH) was first described by Kelly and Wendel [13] in 1991. Since then the surgical technique has been refined to further improve the anatomical and functional outcome.

The current surgical treatment consists of pars plana vitrectomy, induction of a mechanical detachment and removal of the posterior hyaloid, peeling of the epiretinal membranes and of the internal limiting membrane (ILM) with intraocular tamponading using long-acting gas. This technique can achieve MH closure in over 90% of cases. Indeed, in some cases anatomical closure is not obtained (persistent MH) and visual improvement is poor. Moreover, late re-opening of a previously operated MH may occur, with incidences ranging from 9.5% [21] to 4.8% [1].

There may be a variety of reasons for the failure of primary surgery, such as tractions from residual epiretinal membranes, insufficient gas tamponading and poor patient compliance in keeping the prone position, although in most cases there is no obvious cause [3, 21].

2.1.2 Therapeutic Options

So far, the treatment of failed MH (persistent or re-opening MH) is still a challenge for the retinal surgeon. Many therapies have been suggested over time, but in the literature only nonrandomized and noncontrolled studies have been reported, carried out in small anecdotal series. Therefore, at present there is no first-line management and many surgeons give up treatment after one or two attempts at surgery.

Suggested management options have been: observation, laser photocoagulation on the foveal pigment epithelium, and outpatient fluid–gas exchange (FGEX) [2, 11, 19] and surgical retreatment.

2.1.2.1 Observation

Sometimes a MH that has been re-opened late may spontaneously close [7].

2.1.2.2 Laser Photocoagulation and Outpatient FGEX

Laser photocoagulaion and outpatient FGEX was often suggested in the 1990s. Argon laser photocoagulation was applied to the foveal retinal pigment epithelium (RPE) cells in the hole bed; FGEX with 20% sulfur hexafluoride was performed, followed by 2 weeks of prone positioning. Results were encouraging, the procedure was cost-effective, but cataract formation was reported in over 83% of cases [9].

2.1.2.3 Re-Operations

Re-operations have been suggested by many authors including:

2.1.2.3.1 New Vitrectomy Using FGEX and 1,330 ng of Transforming Growth Factor-Beta2

In the 1990s this procedure [8] appeared potentially useful in anecdotal series [15, 26], with success rates ranging from 83 to 100% and cataract incidence ranging from 30 to 90%. Transforming growth factor-beta2 showed a beneficial effect on both neurosensory retinal flattening and visual outcome.

2.1.2.3.2 New Vitrectomy Performing Indocyanine Green-Assisted ILM Peeling and Autologous Platelets Concentrate Application

This procedure has been more recently suggested by the German school: if repeated after the failure of the first surgery for MH it increases the anatomic success rate from 82 to 96% [16].

2.1.2.3.3 New Vitrectomy Using Silicone Oil as Long-Term Endotamponade

Surgical retreatment with silicone oil tamponade avoids prone positioning and can lead to closure of the MH, but often does not achieve good functional results [17, 18, 27]; moreover, the effectiveness of the silicone oil endotamponading of the posterior pole is still debatable [18, 20, 29].

Kokame and Yamamoto [14] have shown that in the upright position a silicone oil bubble does not conform well to the foveal depression and that an interface anterior to the fovea can be observed by OCT. This results in a lack of effective tamponading of the fovea, similar to those observed around the edges of a scleral buckle. The poor tamponading may explain why visual recovery after silicone oil tamponading is poor (Fig. 2.1) [17].

Recently, Satchi and Patel [25] have also visualized the posterior face of the silicone oil bubble with OCT: they have concluded that in eyes that had a silicone fill of over 90%, the silicone oil bubble in the sitting position does not conform to the foveal depression.

2.1.2.3.4 New Vitrectomy Using F6H8

In order to achieve more effective tamponading of the posterior pole, Jonas and Jäger [10] used a heavier-than-water endotamponade, perfluorohexyloctane (F6H8), which is a semifluorinated alkane, in the treatment of recurrent MH. They achieved good anatomical and functional results,

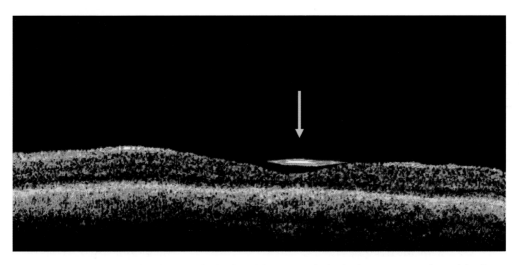

Fig. 2.1 The silicone oil bubble does not fit the foveal depression: lack of effective tamponading of the fovea. *Arrow*: the interface anterior to the foveal depression represents the posterior edge of the silicone bubble

but the incidence of complications (emulsification, epiretinal membrane formation) was significant.

2.1.2.3.5 New Vitrectomy and Endotamponading with HSO (Oxane HD)

We have reported [5, 22, 23] the efficacy and safety of HSO (Oxane HD) as a heavier-than-water endotamponade in the treatment of persistent macular holes, after failure of vitrectomy, ILM peeling, long-acting gas endotamponading, and prone positioning. Oxane HD was removed after 3 months. The main outcome measures were: anatomic success rate (closure of the macular hole) and best corrected visual acuity (BCVA). Anatomic closure of the macular hole was achieved in all patients. Postoperative BCVA improved, ranging from 20/40 to 20/100 with regard to preoperative BCVA ranging from 20/100 to 20/600. In our series OCT images showed that HSO, due to its specific gravity, achieved effective endotamponading of the foveal region in the upright position, allowing a good anatomic and functional recovery (Fig. 2.2). Therefore, HSO can be a safe and effective tool in the treatment of persistent macular hole.

Summary for the Clinician

- The current surgical treatment consists of pars plana vitrectomy, induction of a mechanical detachment and removal of posterior hyaloid, peeling of the epiretinal membranes and of the internal limiting membrane (ILM) with intraocular tamponading using long-acting gas. This technique can achieve MH closure in over 90% of cases.

- Persistent or recurrent macular holes have so far treated by argon laser. Photocoagulation was applied to the foveal retinal pigment epithelium. Transforming growth factor-beta2 showed a beneficial effect on both neurosensory retinal flattening and visual outcome. Silicone oil tamponade avoids prone positioning and can lead to closure of the MH, but often does not achieve good functional results. Autologous platelets concentrate increases the anatomic success rate from 82–96%. Perfluorohexyloctane achieved good anatomical and functional results, but emulsification was significant. Heavier-than-water silicone oil achieved anatomic closure of the macular hole in all patients.

2

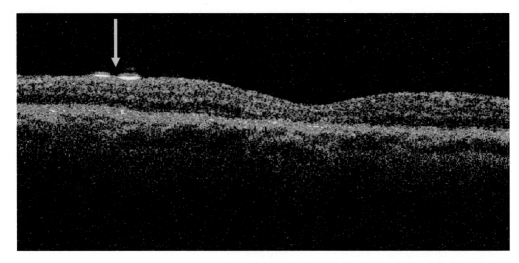

Fig. 2.2 The heavier than water silicone oil (HSO) bubble conforms well with the foveal depression: no prefoveal interface is highlighted. *Arrow*: the interface on the retinal surface represents the posterior edge of the HSO bubble

2.1.3 Rationale of HSO Endotamponading

In our cases, no residual vitreoretinal traction was evident after the initial surgery (Fig. 2.3). The patient's compliance may have been insufficient and postoperative face-down positioning may not have been maintained. Therefore, we decided to use HSO, which did not require any postoperative position and also tamponaded the posterior pole well in the upright position.

As reported in the literature [14], MH closure can also occur without complete tamponading of the central fovea using a silicone oil endotamponade. But, as mentioned above, a prefoveal space can be visualized in silicone-filled eyes. Concentration of growth factors, adjuvants, and indocyanine green in this compartment may influence postoperative visual outcome. On the contrary, OCT images with HSO filling have shown no prefoveal interface. A good tamponading effect is exerted on the foveal region in all patients and achieves MH closure (Fig. 2.4).

The exclusion of the fluid from the surface of the MH may avoid concentration of substance in the foveal region and is critical in favoring the MH seal and preventing epiretinal re-proliferation (Fig. 2.5).

Although Theelen et al. [28] reported increased inflammation in the anterior chamber following endotamponading with HSO over a period of 8 weeks, in our series there were no significant complications due to Oxane HD. The agent is stable [30] and does not emulsify like pure semifluorinated alkanes.

However, at present Densiron, a new HSO, has been made available and fewer side effects have been reported [31]; therefore, we have recently introduced it into the treatment of persistent MH.

2.2 Treatment of Persistent Macular Holes

2.2.1 Heavier Than Water Silicone Oils

Oxane HD (Bausch & Lomb, Toulouse, France) is a heavier-than-water agent with a high specific gravity. It is a mixture of ultra-purified silicone oil (Oxane 5700; Bausch & Lomb) and RMN3, a partially fluorinated and hydrocarbonated olefin. The solution is homogeneous and stable in the presence of water, air or perfluorocarbons. It has a density of 1.02 g/cm^3 and a viscosity of

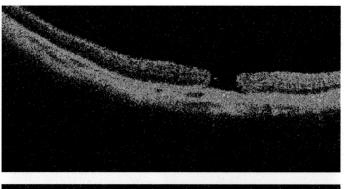

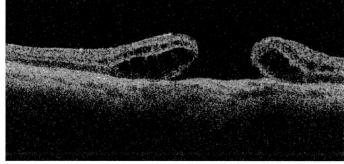

Fig. 2.3 Preoperative optical coherence tomography (OCT) showed a full-thickness macular hole (MH) with elevated margins and no evidence of residual tractions in any patients

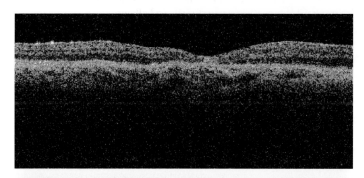

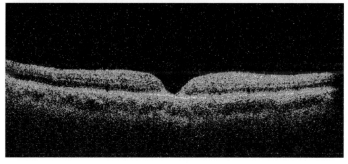

Fig. 2.4 Postoperative OCT showed the anatomic closure of the persistent MH

2

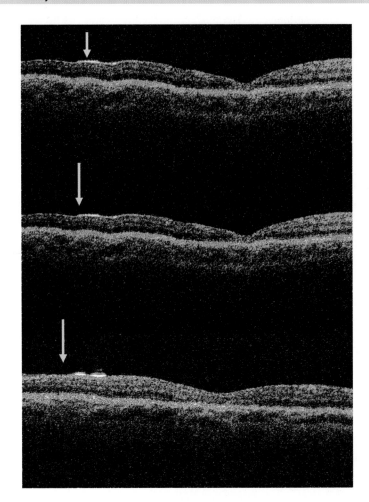

Fig. 2.5 Optical coherence tomography images during endotamponading showed the HSO bubble fitting the foveal profile in all patients

3,300 mPas. Its interfacial tension is higher than 40 mNm.

Densiron-68 (Fluoron) is the other heavier-than-water substance currently used. It is a mixture of Silicone Oil 3000 cs (70%) and F6H8, a semi-fluorinated alkane (30%). This solution is also homogeneous and stable in the presence of water, air or perfluorocarbons. It has a density of 1.06 g/cm³ and a viscosity of 1,400 mPas.

2.2.2 Surgical Technique

Surgery is carried out under regional anesthesia. A standard 20-gauge three-port pars plana vitrectomy is performed. An injection of 0.1 ml of triamcinolone acetonide (4 mg/ml) into the vitreous cavity enhances the visualization of the residual vitreous, in order to achieve complete vitrectomy. If residual hyaloid is evident, the posterior hyaloid membrane is removed after having induced its mechanical detachment.

A solution of indocyanine green (ICG) 0.05% is instilled in order to highlight whether any residual ILM, due to incomplete removal, is still present. The stained residual ILM, if present, is peeled. In order to prevent the contact between the macular hole and the dye, which may be toxic, we routinely use autologous whole blood (AWB) to protect the retinal pigment epithelium [6, 24].

Two milliliters of AWB is taken from a peripheral vein and gently moved to avoid coagulation. 0.1 ml of the AWB is injected into the buffered saline solution-filled vitreous cavity over the posterior pole covers the macular hole. The surplus blood is aspirated with a flute cannula. The blood clot acts as a mechanical barrier on the macular hole and is automatically removed during ILM peeling.

If residual posterior hyaloid or residual ILM is detected intraoperatively, we conclude that the first surgery has been unsuccessful and therefore, after removing all the highlighted tractions, we perform standard long-acting gas endotamponading, followed by prone positioning.

In cases in which the double staining does not enhance any residual and/or newly developed traction, we opt to continue with the HSO endotamponade.

We perform a fluid–air exchange, keeping the globe filled by air for at least 10 min in order to completely dry the vitreous chamber and to achieve complete filling of the globe with the tamponade.

2.2.3 HSO Removal

Heavier than water silicone oil is removed 45–96 days after the initial surgery under regional anesthesia, via a pars plana approach. Under endo-illumination and microscopic visualization, a 19-gauge Teflon tip cannula is held over the optic disc and the HSO is aspirated using the active aspiration of the vitrectomy system. HSO is indeed extremely sticky: this allows good stability, preventing emulsification, but also makes removal quite time-consuming.

2.3 Conclusions

We have shown the sealing of persistent MH under HSOs. As OCT findings have demonstrated, both HSOs – Densiron (Fig. 2.6) and Oxane HD (Fig. 2.7) – are heavier than water, therefore they sink and achieve effective tamponading of the foveal region in the sitting position, allowing a good anatomical and functional recovery.

The surface tension, the specific gravity, and the negative buoyancy of HSOs are much greater than those of standard silicone oil, which is able to support the MH at the beginning at least, when it is open with parafoveal edema and subretinal fluid, but provides less tamponading as soon as the MH closes and the foveal region recovers its normal depression. In the first surgery for idiopathic MH the wettability of standard silicone oil may result in less effective closure with worse visual outcome, but in the treatment of persistent MH it may lead to failure of the treatment.

On the contrary, the behavior of HSOs on the OCT has demonstrated that, thanks to their surface tension and buoyancy, they conform well to the foveal depression with efficient support of the central fovea in the sitting position during the whole sealing process.

Summary for the Clinician

- In our cases the patient's compliance may have been insufficient and postoperative face-down positioning had not been maintained. Therefore, we decided to use HSO, which did not require any postoperative positioning.
- The surgical procedure: standard 20-gauge three-port pars plana vitrectomy. The posterior hyaloid membrane is removed. ICG (0.05%) is instilled. If residual posterior hyaloid or residual ILM is detected intraoperatively, we perform standard long-acting gas endotamponading, followed by prone positioning. If the double staining does not enhance any residual and/or newly developed traction, we decide to continue with the HSO endotamponading.
- Thanks to their surface tension and buoyancy, HSOs conform well to the foveal depression with efficient support of the central fovea in the sitting position during the whole sealing process.

2

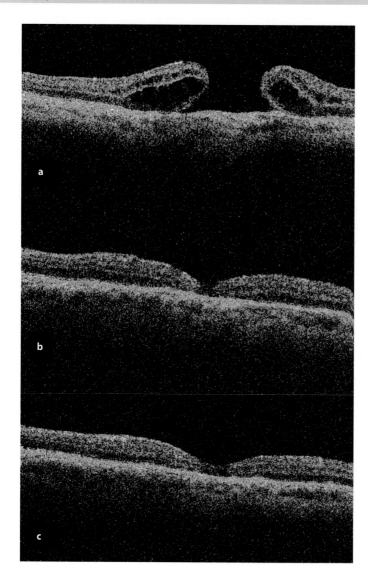

Fig. 2.6 Sealing of persistent MH under HSO (Densiron). **a** Preoperative OCT. **b** One day, **c** 7 days after surgery

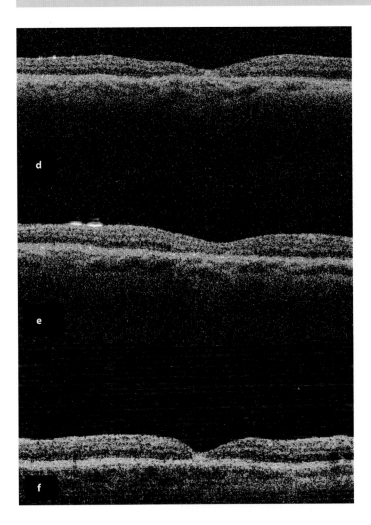

Fig. 2.6 (*Continued*) Sealing of persistent MH under HSO (Densiron). **d** 15 days, **e** 1 month after surgery. **f** After Oxane HD removal

2

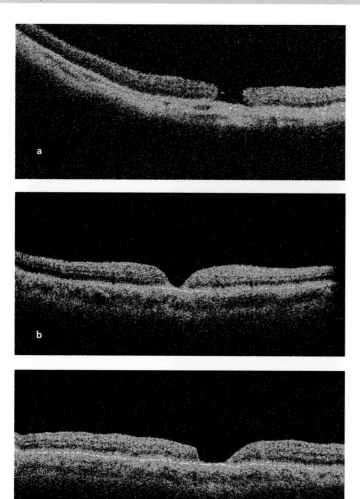

Fig. 2.7 Sealing of persistent MH under HSO (Oxane HD). **a** Preoperative OCT. **b** One day, **c** 7 days after surgery

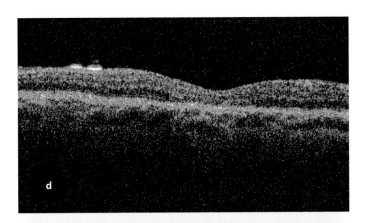

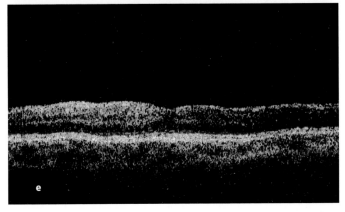

Fig. 2.7 (*Continued*) Sealing of persistent MH under HSO (Oxane HD). **d** 1 month after surgery. **e** After Oxane HD removal

References

1. Cristmas NJ, Smiddy WE, Flynn HW Jr. Reopening of macular holes after initially successful repair. Ophthalmology 1998;105(10):1835–1838.
2. Del Priore LV, Kaplan HJ, Bonham RD. Laser photocoagulation and fluid-gas exchange for recurrent macular hole. Retina 1994;14(4):381–382.
3. Fekrat S, Wendel RT, del la Cruz Z, Green WR. Clinicopathologic correlation of an epiretinal membrane associated with a recurrent macular hole. Retina 1995;15:53–57.
4. Gass JD. Idiopathic senile macular hole: its early stages and pathogenesis. 1988. Retina 2003;23:629–639.
5. Genovesi-Ebert F, Rizzo S, Belting C, Vento A, Cresti F, Martini R, Palla M. Oxane HD as internal tamponade in the treatment of persisting macular holes. Invest. Ophthalmol. Vis. Sci. 2005;46:E-Abstract 5503.
6. Genovesi-Ebert F, Belting C, Di Bartolo E, Vento A, Palla M, Rizzo S. Modified technique for safer indocyanine green-assisted peeling of the retinal internal limiting membrane during vitrectomy surgery for macular hole repair. Invest. Ophthalmol. Vis. Sci. 2003;44:E-Abstract 2987.
7. Gross JC. Late reopening and spontaneous closure of previously repaired macular holes. Am. J. Ophthalmol. 2005;140(3):556–558.
8. Ie D, Glaser BM, Tompson JT, Syaarda RN, Gordon LW. Retreatment of full thickness macular holes persisting after prior vitrectomy. A pilot study. Ophthalmology 1993;100(12):1787–1793.
9. Ikuno Y, Kamei M, Saito Y, Ohji M, Tano Y. Photocoagulation and fluid gas exchange to treat persistent macular holes after vitrectomy. Ophthalmology 1998;105(8):1411
10. Jonas JB, Jäger M. Perfluorohexyloctane endotamponade for treatment of persisting macular hole. Eur. J. Ophthalmol. 2003;13:103–104.
11. Johnson RN, McDonald HR, Schatz H, Ai E. Outpatient postoperative fluid-gas exchange after early failed vitrectomy surgery for macular hole. Ophthalmology 1997;104:2009–2013.
12. Karia N, LaidlawA, West J, et al. Macular hole surgery using silicone oil tamponade. Br. J. Ophthalmol. 2001;85:1320–1323.
13. Kelly NE, Wendel RT. Vitreous surgery for idiopathic macular holes. Results of a pilot study. Arch. Ophthalmol. 1991;109:654–659.
14. Kokame GT, Yamamoto I. Silicone oil versus gas tamponade. Ophthalmology 2004;111:851–852.
15. Kozy DW, Maberley AL. Closure of persistent macular holes with human recombinant transforming factor-beta 2. Can. J. Ophthalmol. 1996;32(4):179–182.
16. Kube T, Hermel M, Dahlke C, Hutschenreuter G, Schrage N, Kirchoff B. Macular hole surgery: experience with autologous platelet concentrate and indocyanine green-assisted internal limiting membrane peeling. Klin. Monatsbl. Augenheilkd. 2002;219(12):883–888.
17. Kumar V, Banerjee S, Loo AV, et al. Macular hole surgery with silicone oil. Eye 2002;16:121–125.
18. Lai JC, Stinnett SS, McCuen BW. Comparison of silicone oil versus gas tamponade in the treatment of idiopathic full-thickness macular hole. Ophthalmology 2003;110:1170–1174.
19. Ohana E, Blumenkranz MS. Treatment of reopened macular hole after vitrectomy by laser and outpatient fluid-gas exchange. Ophthalmology 1998;105:1398–1403.
20. Oz O, Akduman L. Successful surgical repair and good visual outcome of a recurrent macular hole of seven years duration. Eur. J. Ophthalmol. 2003;13(6):588–589.
21. Paques M, Massin P, Blain P, et al. Long-term incidence of reopening of macular holes. Ophthalmology 2000;107:760–765.
22. Rizzo S, Belting C, Genovesi-Ebert F. Two cases of giant retinal tear after implantation of a phakic intraocular lens. Retina 2003;23(3):411–413.
23. Rizzo S, Genovesi-Ebert F, Belting C, Vento A, Cresti F. A pilot study on the use of silicone oil-RMN3 as heavier-than-water endotamponade agent. Graefes Arch Clin. Exp. Ophthalmol. 2005(11):1153–1157.
24. Rizzo S, Belting C, Genovesi-Ebert F, Vento A, Cresti F. Modified technique for a safer indocyanine green-assisted peeling of the internal limiting membrane during vitrectomy for macular hole repair. Graefes Arch. Clin. Exp. Ophthalmol. 2006 May 17; [Epub ahead of print].
25. Satchi K, Patel CK. Posterior chamber compartments demonstrated by optical coherence tomography in silicone filled eyes, following macular hole surgery. Clin. Exp. Ophthalmol. 2005;33(6):619–622.

26. Smiddy WE, Sjaarda RN, Glaser BM, Flynn HW Jr, Thompson JT, Hanham A, Murphy RP. Reoperation after failed macular hole surgery. Retina 1996;16(1):13–18.

27. Tafoya ME, Lambert HM, Vu L, Ding M. Visual outcomes of silicone oil versus gas tamponade for macular hole surgery. Semin. Ophthalmol. 2003;18:127–131.

28. Theelen T, Tilanus MA, Klevering BJ. Intraocular inflammation following endotamponade with high-density silicone oil. Graefes Arch. Clin. Exp. Ophthalmol. 2004;242:617–620.

29. Voo I, Siegner SW, Mall KW. Silicone oil tamponade to seal macular holes. Ophthalmology 2001;108(9):1516–1517.

30. Wolf S, Schon V, Meier P, Wiedemann P. Silicone oil-RMN3 mixture ("heavy silicone oil") as internal tamponade for complicated retinal detachment. Retina 2003;23:335–342.

31. Wong D, Van der Meurs JC, Stappler T, Groenwald C, Pearce IA, Manousakis E, Herbert EN. A pilot study on the use of a perfluorohexyloctane/silicone oil solution as a heavier than water internal tamponade agent. Br. J. Ophthalmol. 2005;89(6):662–665.

Chapter 3

The Role of Combined Adjunctive 5-Fluorouracil and Low Molecular Weight Heparin in Proliferative Vitreoretinopathy Prevention

3

David G. Charteris, D. Wong

Core Messages

■ Investigation of the basic pathological processes of proliferative vitreoretinopathy (PVR) has allowed the rational design of adjunctive treatment regimes to prevent PVR development.

■ The efficacy of the combination of 5-fluorouracil (5FU) and low molecular weight heparin (LMWH) in preventing PVR has been tested in three large-scale randomized clinical trials of vitrectomy surgery.

■ The results of these trials indicate that the 5FU/LMWH combination is effective in preventing PVR in high-risk retinal detachments, but not in unselected cases or in eyes in which there is established PVR.

■ Reduced visual acuity levels suggest that the combination may have a toxic effect in macular-sparing unselected retinal detachments.

3.1 Introduction

Proliferative vitreoretinopathy (PVR) is a process of cellular proliferation and fibrocellular membrane contraction that complicates between 5 and 12% of all retinal detachments [11]. Retinal detachments that develop PVR require more healthcare resources, more operations, and have poorer visual outcomes than retinal detachments that do not develop PVR [23]. Binocular vision outcomes are notably unsatisfactory in patients with PVR [2]. Once PVR has developed visual recovery is often limited despite improved anatomical surgical success rates [20, 21].

Proliferative vitreoretinopathy has a higher incidence in retinal detachments secondary to giant retinal tears (16–41%) and in eyes sustaining penetrating trauma (10–45%, highest in perforating trauma and blunt injuries) [11]. In addition, PVR is an important complication of retinal translocation occurring in between 10 and 18% of eyes [12, 13, 24].

The continued incidence of PVR, the consequences of repeat surgery, and worse visual outcomes have led to a focus on PVR prevention and improving the results of PVR surgery by the use of pharmacological adjunctive agents. A group of researchers in the UK, the PVR Study Group, was established in the mid-1990s to pool knowledge and resources to investigate the clinical potential of adjunctive medication to improve outcomes in retinal detachment and PVR surgery. Subsequently, UK researchers have completed three randomized controlled trials on the use of 5-fluorouracil (5FU) and low molecular weight heparin (LMWH) as adjuncts in the prevention and treatment of PVR. The results of these trials, comprising in total over 970 patients, and the implications for clinical practice are discussed in this chapter.

3.2 PVR Pathobiology

3.2.1 PVR Development

Retinal breaks and subsequent retinal detachment initiates a pathological process that can result in PVR. Blood–retinal barrier breakdown (of which dense vitreous hemorrhage is an extreme form) and release of retinal pigment epithelial (RPE) cells into the vitreous cavity contribute to the process of peri-retinal membrane formation, which may progress to clinical PVR [8]. Separation of the neural retina from the RPE initiates a series of pathological changes, notably upregulation of all non-neural cells and deconstruction and loss of neural components of the retina, which further contribute to PVR development (and are likely to be central to the failure of functional recovery of the retina) [26].

3.2.2 PVR Components

Clinical observation and laboratory investigations undertaken on eyes with PVR and surgically removed specimens have identified potential targets for pharmacological adjuncts (summarized in [7]). The cellular components of PVR peri-retinal membranes (RPE, glial, inflammatory, and fibroblastic cells) proliferate, may also be contractile and are thus targets for antiproliferative agents. Drugs that inhibit cellular or membrane contraction can potentially also play a role in PVR prevention. The formation of fibrin following retinal detachment or vitreoretinal surgery has been linked to PVR development [14] and agents aimed at limiting fibrin formation may reduce PVR. The extracellular matrix is a prominent component in PVR membranes and inhibition of matrix deposition is another potential strategy for PVR treatment. The turnover and remodeling of the extracellular matrix is regulated by matrix metalloproteinases (MMPs) and their natural inhibitors: tissue inhibitors of

metalloproteinases (TIMPs) [25]. Modification of the actions of MMP or TIMPs also has potential in PVR management. Various growth factors/cytokines have been identified in PVR and as manipulation of the growth factor response becomes clinically viable this may be a possible future treatment for PVR prevention.

Summary for the Clinician

- Proliferative vitreoretinopathy remains a clinical problem for vitreoretinal surgeons, occurring in a significant minority of retinal detachments and with a higher incidence in more complex vitreoretinal conditions.
- Surgery for PVR is resource-intensive and outcomes often unsatisfactory.
- Clinical and laboratory investigations have provided important data on the pathogenesis of PVR, which has subsequently aided the design of adjunctive pharmacological strategies for PVR prevention.

3.3 Adjunctive Agents

Various pharmacological adjuncts have been investigated in laboratory studies or in uncontrolled or pilot clinical studies [8, 10]. To date, only daunomycin [30] and a combination of 5FU and LMWH have been the subject of large-scale randomized clinical trials.

3.3.1 5-Fluorouracil

5-Fluorouracil is a synthetic pyrimidine analogue that modifies protein synthesis by binding to and inhibiting the enzyme thymidylate synthetase, and by incorporation into RNA causing coding errors in protein translation, thus inhibiting cellular proliferation. 5FU has been used in the treatment of solid tumors and proliferative dermatological conditions, and in the prevention of scarring following glaucoma surgery. It has been shown to be effective in reducing the incidence of PVR in animal models [5, 28]. Experimental work has demonstrated that short-term exposure to 5FU produces prolonged growth arrest of Tenon's capsule fibroblasts in vitro [17] and of RPE cells in vivo [19], suggesting that transient exposure (for example during vitrectomy surgery) can have prolonged pharmacological effects.

The cellular effect of 5FU could potentially produce intraocular toxicity. Animal experiments did not demonstrate toxicity at lower dosage levels [5, 29], but did show both histological (loss of photoreceptor outer segments, loss of ribosomes) and electrophysiological (loss of b-wave) alterations at higher dose levels [29]. These changes demonstrated only limited recovery and imply caution in the clinical intraocular use of 5FU.

3.3.2 Low Molecular Weight Heparin

Heparin has multiple cellular effects that can potentially inhibit PVR development. It reduces fibrin formation, interferes with cell-substrate adhesion by binding fibronectin, binds fibrogenic growth factors, and inhibits cellular proliferation including scleral fibroblasts and RPE cells [8]. The low molecular weight fragments of heparin have less effect on the coagulation cascade or platelet function, reducing the risk of hemorrhagic complications. Experimental animal studies have demonstrated that LMWH reduces PVR [7] and that it is not toxic in the rabbit eye when infused at a dose of 5 IU/ml [14].

3.3.3 Initial Clinical Studies

A prospective study of eyes undergoing vitrectomy for vitreous hemorrhage or retinal detachment that received 10 mg of 5FU at the completion of surgery [4] demonstrated that this dosage was well tolerated and a previous study of PVR cases did not find any toxicity at a dose level of 1 mg [6]. Both studies had relatively small numbers of patients and neither demonstrated a beneficial effect of the adjunctive 5FU.

A clinical trial investigating the effect of heparin on post-vitrectomy fibrin formation demonstrated a reduction following intravitreal infusion of 10 IU/ml heparin, but an associated increased incidence of intraoperative bleeding [16]. Intravenous and 5 IU/ml infusion of heparin showed a trend toward lower rates of fibrin production and no toxicity.

3.4 Clinical Trials of Combined Adjunctive 5FU and LMWH

The potentially synergistic effects of the combination of 5FU and LMWH on modifying PVR development and clinical outcomes in eyes undergoing vitrectomy surgery have been investigated in three large-scale clinical trials (each given the abbreviated title "PVR"). These investigated:

1. High-risk retinal detachments in eyes undergoing vitrectomy and gas exchange (PVR 1) [3];
2. Established PVR in eyes undergoing vitrectomy and silicone oil exchange (PVR 2) [11];
3. Unselected primary retinal detachments in eyes undergoing vitrectomy and gas exchange (PVR 3; data unpublished).

The same combination of 5FU and LMWH was also used for a consecutive noncomparative series of macular translocation on the basis that this surgery was related to a high rate of retinal detachment and PVR.

3.4.1 Adjunctive Regime

The same adjunctive medication regime was used in the treatment arm of all three trials. 5FU at a concentration of 200 mg/ml and LMWH at a concentration of 5 IU/ml were added to the Hartmann's solution used as the vitrectomy infusion fluid. Plain Hartmann's solution was used in controls. The treatment/placebo solution was used for 1 h during surgery and changed for plain Hartmann's solution if surgery continued beyond this point. Because of the potential teratogenic risk premenopausal women were excluded from all studies.

3.4.2 High-Risk Retinal Detachments in Eyes Undergoing Vitrectomy and Gas Exchange (PVR 1)

To identify patients at a high risk of developing PVR, a regression formula, based on previous analysis of PVR risk factors, was used [19]. The formula is as follows:

Risk of PVR developing = 2.88 × (preoperative grade C PVR) + 1.85 × (preoperative grade B PVR) + 2.92 × (aphakia or pseudophakia without intact posterior capsule) + 1.77 × (anterior uveitis) + 1.23 × (quadrants of detachment) + 0.83 × (vitreous hemorrhage) + 1.23 × (previous cryotherapy)

If a risk factor is present, 1 is added to the equation, for quadrants of detachment 1–4 is added. Using a discriminant rule a total risk factor score of greater than 6.33 defines a retinal detachment as high-risk and less than 6.33 as low-risk. In our study, high-risk cases have been shown to have a postoperative incidence of PVR of 28% and low-risk cases of 9% [18].

Using this formula patients deemed to be at high risk of PVR development were considered for inclusion in the trial. Those who had had previous vitrectomy were excluded and those who had undergone previous scleral buckling (10–15% of the treatment and placebo groups) were included.

A total of 174 patients were recruited. Internal tamponade was achieved using SF6 gas in approximately 50%, C3F8 gas in 41–46%, and unplanned use of silicone oil was carried out in 3–8% of patients. The incidence of postoperative PVR was significantly lower in the treatment group (12.6%) than in the placebo group (26.4%; $p=0.02$). Patients in the placebo group had significantly worse final visual acuity ($p=0.048$) and showed a trend toward more re-operations resulting from PVR. The total numbers of primary successes and patients undergoing re-operation did not appear to be influenced by the treatment regime. Complication rates were low and evenly distributed between the two groups. The high rates of PVR in the patient groups in this trial were considered to be due to the selection of higher risk cases based on the risk formula. On the basis of the results of this study the treatment regime appeared safe and it was recommended that it would reduce PVR rates in high-risk retinal detachments.

3.4.3 Established PVR in Eyes Undergoing Vitrectomy and Silicone Oil Exchange (PVR 2)

Patients with retinal detachment who had developed PVR grade C or greater (anterior or posterior) [22] and who were to undergo vitrectomy and silicone oil exchange were recruited. A total of 157 patients were randomized to surgery with or without adjunctive 5FU and LMWH. Forty-five to fifty patients had not had previous vitreoretinal surgery. There were no significant differences in primary (retinal re-attachment without further vitreoretinal intervention at 6 months) or secondary (complete or posterior retinal re-attachment, visual acuity, hypotony, cataract, keratopathy) outcome measures although there was a lower incidence of macular pucker in the treatment group that marginally failed to reach statistical significance ($p=0.068$). No toxic effects of the adjunctive treatment were observed. Based on these results adjunctive 5FU and LMWH was not recommended for cases of established PVR.

3.4.4 Unselected Primary Retinal Detachments in Eyes Undergoing Vitrectomy and Gas Exchange (PVR 3)

The increasing trend toward managing rhegmatogenous retinal detachment by primary vitrectomy and the positive result of the use of adjunctive 5FU and LMWH in high-risk retinal detachments raised the question of whether the treatment regime should be used in all primary vitrectomy operations for retinal detachment. Because of the high primary success rate of retinal detachment repair and the relatively low rate of PVR, a much higher sample size was required and 641 patients were recruited into a randomized controlled trial at Moorfields Eye Hospital, London and St Paul's Eye Unit, Liverpool. These have now completed 6 months' follow-up.

The overall primary success rate of surgery was 84.4% and the complete anatomical attachment rate at 6 months was 98%. There was no significant difference in the rate of PVR – in the treatment group 7% developed PVR compared with 4.9% in the placebo group, or in mean final visual acuity. Notably, in patients with macular sparing retinal detachments the final visual acuity was significantly worse, raising the possibility of a toxicity effect of the adjunctive medications.

3.4.5 Macular Translocation with 360° Retinotomy

This surgery is at a high risk of causing proliferative vitreoretinopathy. In the first 7 cases reported by Wolf et al., 3 patients had retinal detachment and another patient had macular pucker [32]. The largest report case series was from Cologne and involved 90 patients. The retinal detachment rate was 19% (95% CI between 11–29%) [1]. The case series from Antwerp had a high success rate in terms of visual improvement; there was a retinal detachment and PVR rate of 18% (95% CI between 9 and 31%) [24]. In Liverpool, 100 consecutive cases of macular translocation were carried out using 5FU and LMWH. The initial experience was positive. Retinal detachment occurred in 3 of the first 29 patients (95% CI between 2 and 27%) [33]. Subsequent audit of the first 63 patients with a minimum follow-up of 2 years from the same case series revealed 8 cases of retinal detachment giving a rate of 13% (95% CI between 6 and 24%) [27]. It is not possible to draw any valid conclusions without a randomized trial, as the rate of retinal detachment depended not only on PVR, but also on other surgical factors including the learning curve [30].

3.5 Implications for Clinical Use

3.5.1 Uncomplicated Primary Retinal Detachments

On the basis of the large-scale trial outlined above (PVR3), it is recommended that 5FU and LMWH should not be routinely used in primary retinal detachment repair. Because of the possible toxic effect of the adjunctive medications highlighted by the reduced visual acuity in the treatment group when the macula was not involved, caution should be exercised in their use in other situations.

3.5.2 Established PVR

Combined 5FU and LMWH does not improve the outcome of surgery for established PVR. Previous work has demonstrated that daunomycin reduces the rate of re-operations in established PVR [31] and clinicians may consider its use as a per-operative adjunct.

3.5.3 High-Risk Retinal Detachments

High-risk retinal detachment cases, identified by a risk factor formula and possibly selected by clinicians on the basis of clinical experience, should be considered for adjunctive 5FU and LMWH as a per-operative infusion in vitrectomy surgery.

3.5.4 Intraocular Trauma Patients Undergoing Vitrectomy Surgery

There is a significant risk of PVR development following intraocular trauma. Many of the risk factors in trauma are analogous to those identified in high-risk retinal detachments – extensive blood–retinal barrier breakdown, intraocular inflammation, and RPE cell dispersion. Clinicians may therefore elect to extrapolate the results of the use of 5FU and LMWH in high-risk retinal detachments to trauma cases in patients undergoing vitrectomy. It should be noted, however, that there are unresolved toxicity issues relating to trauma cases, for example the use of LMWH in eyes that may already be predisposed to hemorrhage.

Summary for the Clinician

- The use of a preoperative combined adjunctive regime of 5FU and LMWH to prevent PVR or recurrent PVR following retinal detachment has now been investigated in three large, prospective, randomized, controlled trials.
- These have demonstrated improved results in high-risk retinal detachments, but no benefit in unselected primary detachments or established PVR.
- Reduced visual acuity was observed in unselected macula-sparing retinal detachments receiving the adjuncts and may be due to a toxic effect.

References

1. Aisenbrey S, Lafaut BA, Szurman P, Grisanti S, Luke C, Krott R, et al. Macular translocation with 360 degrees retinotomy for exudative age-related macular degeneration. Arch Ophthalmol 2002;120(4):451–459.
2. Andenmatten R, Gonvers M. Sophisticated vitreoretinal surgery in patients with a healthy fellow eye. Graefes Arch Ophthalmol 1993;231:495–499.
3. Asaria RHY, Kon CH, Bunce C, Charteris DG, Wong D, Khaw PT, Aylward GW. Adjuvant 5-fluorouracil and heparin prevents proliferative vitreoretinopathy: results from a randomized, double-blind, controlled clinical trial. Ophthalmology 2001;108:1179–1183.
4. Blankenship GW. Evaluation of a single intravitreal injection of 5-fluorouracil in vitrectomy cases. Graefes Arch Clin Exp Ophthalmol 1989;227(6):565–568.
5. Blumenkranz MS, Ophir A, Claflin AJ, Hajek A. Fluorouracil for the treatment of massive periretinal proliferation. Am J Ophthalmol 1982;94:458–467.
6. Blumenkranz M, Hernandez E, Ophir A, Norton E. 5-fluorouracil: new applications in complicated retinal detachment for an established antimetabolite. Ophthalmology 1984;91:122–130.
7. Blumenkranz MS, Hartzer MK, Iverson D. An overview of potential applications of heparin in vitreoretinal surgery. Retina 1992;12 (3 Suppl): S71–S74.
8. Charteris DG. Proliferative vitreoretinopathy: pathobiology, surgical management and adjunctive treatment. Br J Ophthalmol 1995;79:953–960.
9. Charteris DG. Surgery for proliferative vitreoretinopathy. In: Evidence based ophthalmology, eds. Wormald, Seeth & Henshaw. BMJ, London 2004.
10. Charteris DG, Sethi CS, Lewis GP, Fisher SK. Proliferative vitreoretinopathy – developments in adjunctive treatment and retinal pathology. Eye 2002;16:369–374.
11. Charteris DG, Aylward GW, Wong D, Groenewald C, Asaria RHY, Bunce C. A randomised controlled trial of combined 5-fluorouracil and low molecular weight heparin in management of established proliferative vitreoretinopathy. Ophthalmology. 2004 111:2240–2245.
12. Eckardt C, Eckardt U, Conrad H-G. Macular rotation with and without counter-rotation of the globe in patients with age-related macular degeneration. Graefes Arch Clin Exp Ophthalmol 1999;237:313–325.
13. Fujii GY, Pieramici DJ, Humayun MS, Schachat AP, Reynolds SM, Melia M, DeJuan E. Complications associated with limited macular translocation. Am J Ophthalmol 2000;130:751–762.
14. Iverson DA, Katsura H, Hartzer MK, Blumenkranz MS. Inhibition of intraocular fibrin formation following infusion of low-molecular-weight heparin during vitrectomy. Arch Ophthalmol 1991;109(3):405–409.
15. Jaffe GF, Schwartz D, Han DP, Gottlieb M Hartz A, McCarthy D, Mi WF, Abrams GW. Risk factors for postvitrectomy fibrin formation. Am J Ophthalmol 1990;109:661–667.
16. Johnson RN, Blankenship G. A prospective randomised clinical trial of heparin therapy for postoperative intraocular fibrin. Ophthalmology 1988;95:312–317.
17. Khaw PT, Sherwood MB, MacKay SL, et al. Five-minute treatments fluorouracil, floxuridine and mitomycin have long-term effects on human Tenon's capsule fibroblasts. Arch Ophthalmol 1992;110:1150–1154

18. Kon CH, Occleston NL, Foss A, Sheridan C, Aylward GW, Khaw PT. Effects of single, short-term exposures of human retinal pigment epithelial cells to thiotepa or 5-fluorouracil: implications for the treatment of proliferative vitreoretinopathy. Br J Ophthalmol 1998;82(5):554–560.

19. Kon CH, Asaria RH, Occleston NL, Khaw PT, Aylward GW. Risk factors for proliferative vitreoretinopathy after primary vitrectomy: a prospective study. Br J Ophthalmol 2000;84:506–511.

20. Lewis H, Aaberg TM. Causes of failure after repeat vitreoretinal surgery for recurrent proliferative vitreoretinopathy. Am J Ophthalmol 1991;111:15–19.

21. Lewis H, Aaberg TM, Abrams GW. Causes of failure after initial vitreoretinal surgery for severe proliferative vitreoretinopathy. Am J Ophthalmol 1991;111:8–14.

22. Machemer R, Aaberg TM, Freeman HM, et al. An updated classification of retinal detachment with proliferative vitreoretinopathy. Am J Ophthalmol 1991;112:159–165.

23. Patel NN, Bunce C, Asaria RH, Charteris DG. Resources involved in managing retinal detachment complicated by proliferative vitreoretinopathy (PVR). Retina 2004;24:883–887.

24. Pertile G, Claes C. Macular translocation with 360 degree retinotomy for management of age-related macular degeneration with subfoveal choroidal neovascularisation. Am J Ophthalmol 2002;134:560–565.

25. Salzmann J, Limb A, Khaw PT, Gregor ZJ, Webster L, Chignell AH, Charteris DG. Matrix metalloproteinases and their natural inhibitors in fibrovascular membranes of proliferative diabetic retinopathy. Br J Ophthalmol 2000;84:1090–1096.

26. Sethi CS, Lewis GP, Fisher SK, Leitner WP, Mann DL, Luthert PJ, Charteris DG. Glial remodelling and neural plasticity in human retinal detachment with proliferative vitreoretinopathy. Invest Ophthalmol Vis Sci 2005 46:329–342.

27. Stappler T, Wong D. Does it work? A longitudinal and comparative study of eyes with exudative AMD treated with 360° macular translocation using the fellow eye as control. Abstract. Invest Ophthalmol Vis Sci. 2005;46:3628.

28. Stern WH, Guerin CJ, Erickson PA, Lewis GP, Anderson DH, Fisher SK. Ocular toxicity of fluorouracil after vitrectomy. Am J Ophthalmol 1983;96(1):43–51.

29. Stern WH, Lewis GP, Erickson PA, Guerin CJ, Anderson DH, Fisher SK, et al. Fluorouracil therapy for proliferative vitreoretinopathy after vitrectomy. Am J Ophthalmol 1983;96(1):33–42.

30. Toth CA, Freedman SF. Macular translocation with 360-degree peripheral retinectomy impact of technique and surgical experience on visual outcomes. Retina 2001;21(4):293–303.

31. Wiedemann P, Hilgers RD, Bauer P, Heimann K. Adjunctive daunorubicin in the treatment of proliferative vitreoretinopathy: results of a multicenter clinical trial. Am J Ophthalmol 1998;126:550–559.

32. Wolf S, Lappas A, Weinberger AW, Kirchhof B. Macular translocation for surgical management of subfoveal choroidal neovascularizations in patients with AMD: first results. Graefes Arch Clin Exp Ophthalmol 1999;237(1):51–57.

33. Wong D, Stanga P, Briggs M, Lenfestey P, Lancaster E, Li KK, et al. Case selection in macular relocation surgery for age related macular degeneration. Br J Ophthalmol 2004;88(2):186–190.

Slippage of the Retina: What Causes It and How Can It Be Prevented?

4

David Wong

Core Messages

- Slippage is the posterior displacement of aqueous underneath the retina caused by an incoming bubble of endotamponade.
- It occurs during the exchange of pre-retinal fluid with air or silicone oil.
- It occurs more readily when fluid is exchanged for air rather than silicone oil.
- It occurs with large breaks, giant retinal tears, and 360° retinotomies (as in macular translocation surgery).
- It is possible to achieve a successful fluid exchange procedure without slippage by exchanging perfluorocarbon liquids with silicone or air.
- Prevention of slippage is reliant on the complete and meticulous elimination of aqueous, not just from the vitreous cavity, but also from the infusion tubing and the three-way taps.

4.1 Introduction

This chapter deals not only with slippage, but also with the various means of exchanging fluids inside the eye. The author has been involved in devising a form of surgery for limited translocation [1] in which slippage was an important complication to avoid. Latterly, I have had experience of over 100 cases of full macular translocation with 360° retinotomy [2, 3]. Additionally, the management of complex proliferative vitreoretinopathy cases often involves the use of retinotomies [4]. The treatment of these and cases of giant retinal

tears has prompted me to study the phenomenon of slippage using a model eye chamber [5]. It is hoped that readers of this chapter gain some insight into the interaction of endotamponade and aqueous inside the vitreous cavity.

4.2 What is Slippage?

Slippage is the posterior displacement of fluid underneath the retina. It occurs during the fluid exchange procedure and is caused by an incoming bubble of endotamponade such as air or silicone oil. Slippage can result in the following:

1. Subretinal fluid will be loculated around the posterior pole.
2. The peripheral retinal edge of a giant retinal tear will be displaced posteriorly.
3. This will in turn leave an area of exposed retinal pigment epithelium and may increase the tendency toward proliferative vitreoretinopathy or hypotony.
4. In the case of 360° retinotomy, slippage can give rise to retinal folds.

It is therefore desirable to avoid these complications. To do this, it is necessary to understand how slippage occurs. Interfacial tensions between different liquids and to a lesser extent, the specific gravity of endotamponade agents are relevant.

4.2.1 Surface Tension and Interfacial Tension

When two immiscible fluids come into contact with one another an interface is formed. One of the immiscible fluids could for example be air and the other water. Figure 4.1 illustrates a droplet of water at the tip of a pipette. A molecule "I" at the centre of the droplet is attracted in all directions to every other molecule inside the droplet, whereas a molecule "S" at the surface has a net attraction inwards. Surface tension is the van de Waals attractive force between the molecules

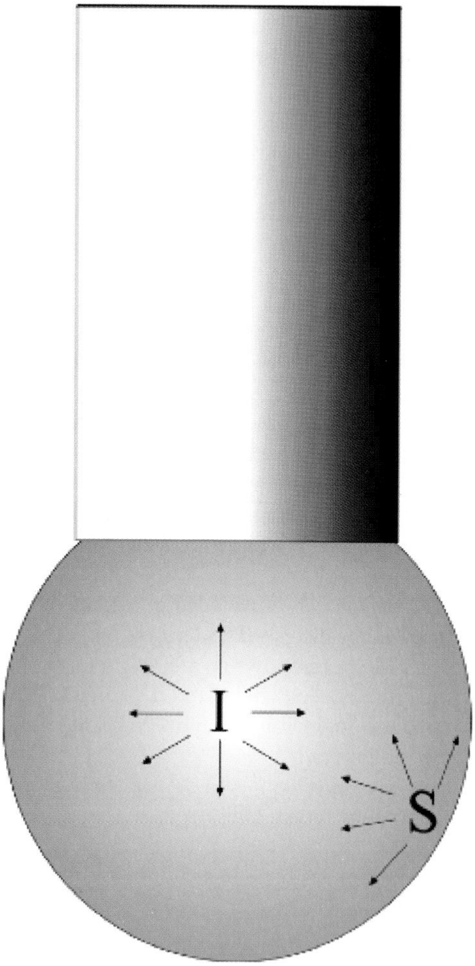

Fig. 4.1 Droplet of water at the end of a pipette. A molecule of water situated inside the droplet at "I" is attracted to its surrounding molecules by Van de Waal's forces equally in all directions. A molecule on the surface at "S" would have more attractive forces inside rather than outside such that the resultant force is inwards. Surface tension therefore acts like a 'tight skin' trying to achieve the smallest surface area for a given volume

on the surface of the droplet. This force will tend to minimize the area of the surface.

Surface tension generally refers to the energy between a liquid and air. A more general term is "interfacial energy" and this can be applied to situations when two or more phases are in contact with each other. For example, when perfluorocarbon liquids (PFCL) are used in the eye cavity, three phases are in contact with each another, namely between the retina and the PFCL, between the PFCL and aqueous, and lastly between the aqueous and the retina [6].

As can be seen later, when air or silicone oil is exchanged for the PFCL, a fourth phase is introduced.

4.2.2 Shape of Endotamponade Bubble

The shape of an intraocular bubble depends primarily on the specific gravity of the endotamponade agent and its interfacial tension with water. Air (and all other intraocular gases that we use for surgery) has a high interfacial tension of around 70 mN/m at room temperature; the perfluorocarbon liquids have an intermediate interfacial tension against water of around 50 mN/m, and silicone oil has a relatively low interfacial tension of 36 mN/m [7]. From what we alluded to previously, we would expect a bubble of air (with the highest interfacial tension against water) to be very rounded. Similarly, a bubble of PFCL might be expected to be more rounded than a bubble of silicone oil in water. This clearly is not the case. What we have not taken into account is the influence of buoyancy [8].

Inside an aqueous-filled compartment such as the vitreous cavity of the eye, a bubble of air would float. The specific gravity of gas is of the order of 0.001 g/cm³. Buoyancy is therefore very high and acts on the molecules inside the bubble such that each wants to move upwards. The result is that the bubble is virtually "D" shaped (or more correctly described as a spherical cap) with a flat bottom. Silicone on the other hand, has a specific gravity of 0.97 g/cm³. It is so close to water that a bubble inside it would be almost spherical. PFCL bubbles have an intermediate shape; the bubble is dome-shaped on the top surface [9]. Figure 4.2A is a nuclear magnetic resonance image of an ex vivo porcine eye with an air bubble inside and Fig. 4.2B the same with a bubble of silicone oil inside. Note the air bubble has the shape of a spherical cap and the oil bubble has a more rounded contour.

4.2.3 Surface Property of the Retina

In the past, we have studied the contact angles between bubbles of various tamponade agents against the retina. We found the retina to be highly hydrophilic [6]. This is an important fact and a key to understanding the behavior of fluids inside the eye.

When we alluded to an air bubble in the eye, we said that it has a "D" shape with a flat bottom. What happens at the edge? There is a meniscus, and its shape is convex downward. One simple consideration is to note that the interfacial tension between water and air is high, so that is why the meniscus is convex. In practice, the situation is more complex. At the meniscus, three phases are in contact with one another, namely air against retina, retina against water, water against air. Because the retina is highly hydrophilic, it prefers to be in touch with water rather than with air, hence the shape of the meniscus.

The situation regarding PFCL is similar. It has a moderately high interfacial tension against water. The retina, being hydrophilic, prefers to be in contact with water than with the PFCL. Thus, one can predict that the meniscus will once again be convex; upward this time as PFCL is heavier than water. The top surface of the PFCL is dome-shaped and there is a rim of aqueous around the bubble at the meniscus. This plays an important part in the process of slippage.

4.2.4 Fluid–Air Exchange

To understand how slippage occurs, we first need to consider what happens during a normal fluid–air exchange procedure. Let us suppose that there is rhegmatogenous retinal detachment and there is a posterior retinal break through which subretinal fluid is drained via a flute needle during a three-port pars plana vitrectomy. Air is introduced with a continuous air pump via the infusion port. As the air comes into the eye, the bubble quickly gets larger and adopts its usual D-shape. The pre-retinal fluid is displaced posteriorly and the retina is displaced laterally and becomes attached [10].

Summary for the Clinician

■ The retina is hydrophilic. All intraocular bubbles of endotamponade have a convex meniscus.
■ The shape of intraocular bubbles is determined by chiefly by buoyancy.
■ Air has a very low specific gravity and air bubbles tend to have the shape of a spherical cap (a "D" on its side).
■ Perfluorocarbon liquid bubbles tend to have a dome shape.
■ As air enters the eye, fluid is displaced posteriorly and the retina is displaced laterally.

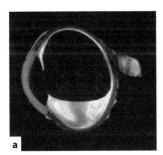 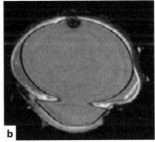

Fig. 4.2 a Nuclear magnetic resonance image of an ex vivo pig's eye with an intraocular bubble of air. Note that the bubble has a relatively flat bottom surface. **b** Similar image with the eye filled with silicone oil. Note the silicone is very rounded in shape

4.3 Setting the Scene for Slippage

During an air–fluid exchange, fluid is displaced posteriorly and the retina is displaced laterally. If the retinal break is not in the posterior pole, then the drainage of pre-retinal fluid before the complete drainage of subretinal fluid can give rise to loculation of fluid posteriorly. This is of little consequence from the point of view of retinal re-attachment, as complete drainage of subretinal fluid is not essential for the successful repair of the retinal detachment, so long as the retinal break is closed. Postoperatively, the subretinal retinal fluid will be absorbed and the retinal pigment epithelium will pump the retina flat [10].

The loculation of subretinal fluid posteriorly, however, exerts a pull on the anterior retina. This can cause one of three effects:

1. The retina can be stretched. This stretching is part of the principle behind macular translocation surgery. Although scleral imbrication has been suggested as a means of generating redundancy [11], doubts have arisen as to whether any redundancy has been achieved [12]. What is certain is that macular translocation can be achieved without scleral buckling just by using a bubble alone—a phenomenon that we referred to in the past as "redistribution of the neurosensory retina" [1, 13]. This simply says the retina has been stretched or compressed.

2. The retina can fold. If there was a substantial amount of residual subretinal fluid and a large bubble was used, then posterior arcuate retinal folds could form postoperatively. These iatrogenic retinal folds often pass through the macula and cause reduction in visual acuity, often accompanied by disturbing symptoms of distortion. This complication is therefore a direct result of drainage technique and has been well reported [14–16]. These iatrogenic folds are not so benign. Untreated, they do not generally "resolve" by remodeling. There was an experimental model in the dog that demonstrated that the outer retinal elements within the fold undergo apoptosis [17]. These iatrogenic folds can be treated by re-detachment of the retina with a subretinal infusion, preferably over a large area and using internal tamponade agents such as gas, PFCL or perfluorohexyloctane [18]. Figure 4.3 shows the pre- and postoperative appearance of an iatrogenic fold successfully treated in this manner.

3. The retina can slip. If the retina is not attached anteriorly, as in the case of a giant retinal tear or extensive circumferential retinotomy, the retina can slip posteriorly leaving a large area of bare retinal pigment epithelium.

Summary for the Clinician

- Incomplete drainage of subretinal fluid in the presence of a large gas bubble can cause stretching of the retina, retinal folds or slippage.
- Limited macular translocation depends on the stretching of the retina.
- Iatrogenic folds passing through the macula can be treated by re-detaching the retina and using air, PFCL or perfluorohexyloctane.
- Perfluorocarbon liquids displaced the subretinal fluid anteriorly. Drainage of the subretinal fluid is often incomplete. Subretinal fluid is loculated anterior to the retinal break and has the shape of a doughnut.

4.3.1 Perfluorocarbon Liquids and the "Doughnut" of Fluid

Perfluorocarbon liquids are sometimes used for the drainage of subretinal fluid. The PFCL is introduced into the vitreous cavity and subretinal fluid is displaced anteriorly. When the fill extends to cover the retinal break, no further drainage of subretinal fluid is possible and the residual subretinal fluid is displaced anteriorly to form a rim of detached retina. The annulus of subretinal fluid is like a doughnut in shape. When PFCL is exchanged for air, the subretinal fluid is displaced backward toward the posterior pole. Those who wish to use PFCL in macula-on retinal detachment in an attempt to prevent iatrogenic detachment of the macula are often disappointed. The doughnut of subretinal fluid displaced posteriorly will detach the macula.

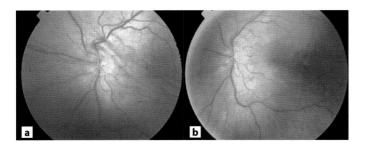

Fig. 4.3 a Fundus color photograph of a retina with an iatrogenic retinal fold. **b** Same fundus after re-detachment of the retina, injection, and subsequent removal of the heavy liquids

One way of preventing macula detachment during a fluid–air exchange procedure is to drain via a relatively posterior iatrogenic drainage retinotomy (or with a flute needle with a flexible drainage tubing that can be advanced under the retina from a peripheral retinal break). Some surgeons prefer an air exchange with a large bubble of PFCL in situ. The PFCL displaces the subretinal fluid anteriorly and the air displaces the subretinal fluid posteriorly. The doughnut of subretinal fluid is at the interface. With indentation and message, the subretinal fluid can be evacuated more completely via a peripheral break. This technique is technically challenging and visualization can be difficult. A simple alternative is, of course, not to perform a complete fluid air exchange. The bubble only needs to be large enough to close the retinal break. A slightly expansile concentration of gas can also be used. Postoperatively, the residual subretinal fluid can be evacuated either with a stream-rolling type procedure of posturing the patient first on one side, then face down, and finally on the other side. It is worth remembering that the aim

of retinal detachment surgery is not the drainage of subretinal fluid, but the closure of retinal breaks. It is not necessary to drain the retina until it is completely flat, certainly not at the expense of detaching the macula in the process.

In the case of a retinal detachment from a giant retinal tear, the doughnut of fluid is still present. The bubble of PFCL has a dome shape and the retinal edge will follow the contour of the endotamponade. When an air–PFCL exchange takes place, the flat bottom surface of the air bubble will displace the doughnut of fluid backward (Fig. 4.4). Because the anterior edge of the giant retinal tear follows the contour of the bubble, the doughnut of fluid will be under the retina. As the air exchange continues, the subretinal fluid will be loculated around the posterior pole. This in turn will stretch the anterior edge of the retina and cause it to be displaced posteriorly; thus, slippage ensues.

In their original paper describing the use of PFCL for giant retinal tears Chang et al. emphasized the need to dry the retinal edge thoroughly. In practice this can be difficult [19]. The process

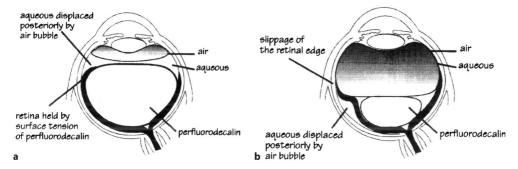

Fig. 4.4 Air/perfluorocarbon liquids (PFCL) exchange procedure during the treatment of a giant retinal tear. **a** Edge of the giant retinal tear following the dome-shaped contours of the PFCL bubble. The air bubble introduced into the eye has a relatively flat bottom surface. **b** Flat bottom surface of the air bubble and the interfacial tension displacing the aqueous posteriorly and external to the retina, which forms a fold ahead of the incoming bubble

4

needs a wide-angle viewing system and is easier if the patient is pseudophakic (or aphakic). To achieve a successful exchange without slippage, it is clearly necessary to gain access and to remove the doughnut of fluid anteriorly. This rim of aqueous is difficult to see as it is at the periphery and at the anterior part of the vitreous cavity; it is situated at the limit of what can be visualized by most viewing systems. A similar approach has been advocated by Han et al. [20].

4.3.2 Seeing and Doing

Wide-angle viewing systems are needed to visualize the doughnut of fluid at the anterior edge of the PFCL bubble. There is a natural tendency to tilt or rotate the eyeball in order to see the periphery. This is a mistake. By tilting the eye, the periphery becomes the dependent (the lowest part). The PFCL will come to occupy this part of the vitreous cavity that can be viewed and the aqueous in fact moved to the upper most part of the eye out of the sight of the surgeon. It is important to remind oneself to keep the eyeball in the primary position. The PFCL bubble inside the eye is like a spirit level; rotating the eye will not help.

External indentation does not help either. It also has a tendency to displace the aqueous. The indent opposes the edge of the giant retinal tear to the retinal pigment epithelium and gives a false impression that there is no residual aqueous present.

Not all wide-angle viewing systems are the same. The non-contact systems such as the EIBOS [21] and BIOM [22] have optional lenses for extra-wide viewing. Contact lens systems in general, however, give wider angle of viewing, allowing better access to pre-equatorial regions of the fundus without tilting the eye. Even so, the view is often not perfect. One is working at the edge of the viewing system and thus there are optical aberrations. The view of a vitreous cavity partly filled with air can be difficult. Air bubbles that are small assume a more spherical shape, giving rise to highly curved and toric refractive surfaces. There may be multiple interfaces that cause specular reflection. The exact interface between PFCL and aqueous may be difficult to discern. The doughnut can be very difficult to see indeed.

It has been pointed out that the oldest wide-angle viewing system is indeed indirect ophthalmoscopy. Those who are skilled in using the indirect ophthalmoscope during vitrectomy may prefer to use it instead of the operating microscope for this stage of the operation.

Equally, evacuation of this aqueous can be difficult simply because the view is not good. The only landmark is the anterior edge of the giant retinal tear. The tip of the aspirating flute needle should be placed just anterior to this. Placing a needle in an eye so far anteriorly runs a high risk of touching the crystalline lens. Clearly the needle should not go across the anterior vitreous cavity. The sclerotomy on the side of the giant retinal tear should be used to introduce the flute needle. Some advocate the routine removal of the clear lens (with or without combined lens implant); others prefer to keep the eye phakic.

Summary for the Clinician

- To visualize the periphery where the doughnut of fluid is situated, it is important to keep the eye in the primary position and take full advantage of the wide-angle optics to see and to aspirate the aqueous anterior to the PFCL bubble. Remember the spirit level. Rotating the eye does not help!
- The manipulation is very close to the lens. In the phakic patient one has to be careful not to touch the lens.
- Overfilling avoids this complicated maneuver (see below).

4.3.3 Air Versus Silicone Oil Exchange for PFCL

It has been noted that slippage does not occur so readily when a direct silicone oil/PFCL exchange is used (instead of first exchanging the PFCL for air and then injecting silicone oil) [23]. When silicone oil is exchanged for PFCL, there are two endotamponades inside the vitreous cavity and four phases in contact with one another. The situation is very complicated, as with four phases there are multiple interfaces, namely: silicone/

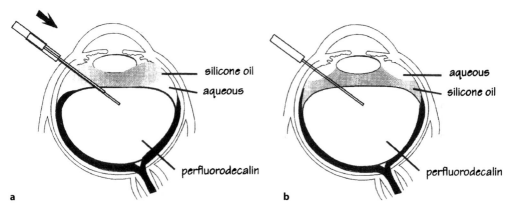

Fig. 4.5 Procedure of silicone oil/PFCL exchange. **a** The edge of the giant retinal tear once again rests on top of the dome-shaped PFCL bubble. The figure shows how a draining flute needle is passed between the silicone oil and the PFCL. Once contact is made the situation in **b** prevails. The interfacial energies of oil and PFCL are such that they prefer to be in contact with one another to the exclusion of the aqueous. At the end of the exchange, we have the anomalous situation of the aqueous being displaced temporally and external to the silicone oil bubble. In this situation, the aqueous escapes via the sclerotomy. Slippage of the retina is much less likely to occur

PFCL, silicone/retina, silicone/aqueous, PFCL/retina, PFCL/aqueous, and retina/aqueous. There are also multiple refractive and specular surfaces such that visualization per-operatively can be difficult and it is difficult to appreciate the interactions among the different fluids. For this reason, we have opted in the past to study this using a transparent eye model chamber.

When silicone is exchanged for PFCL, the important interaction is between these two liquids. Both silicone and PFCL are relatively hydrophobic. The surface energy is lowest when the two liquids are in contact with each other. The two liquids as it were "prefer" to be in contact at the exclusion of aqueous. We have demonstrated in the model eye that passing a flute needle from the silicone into the heavy liquid would make the initial contact between the two. Once this happens, they form an interface at the expense of aqueous (Fig. 4.5).

4.3.4 Oil on Water? No, Water on Oil!

In the model eye, once the oil is introduced and contact is made between the silicone and PFCL, the aqueous is displaced laterally and "above" the silicone oil. This is a phenomenon that we did not visualize clinically. Conceptually, we think

that silicone, being the lightest, would float on top of any residual aqueous in the vitreous cavity. In fact, the specific gravity of silicone is very close to that of water, being $0.97\ g/cm^3$. The aqueous in the vitreous cavity is close to $1.0\ g/cm^3$. The buoyancy force is dependent on the difference in specific gravities between the silicone and the aqueous. The buoyancy was not sufficient to overcome the interfacial energy between the silicone and PFCL. The aqueous in the model chamber was displaced laterally and above the silicone oil, instead of being displaced posteriorly. Slippage therefore does not occur.

Summary for the Clinician

- There is a physical reason why slippage occurs less readily with a silicone oil/PFCL exchange compared with an air/PFCL exchange.
- The buoyancy force of silicone is not sufficient to overcome the interfacial energy between the silicone oil and PFCL.
- Contact between silicone and PFCL excludes aqueous from the interface. The aqueous is displaced laterally and above the oil.

4

4.4 Overfilling and Complete Elimination of Aqueous

We have already established that eliminating the doughnut of aqueous during an air/PFCL exchange can be difficult. It is difficult both in terms of visualization and manipulation. Essentially, one is trying to see and work on one of the most inaccessible parts of the eye.

The alternative involves two separate considerations: overfilling the eye with PFCL and elimination of all aqueous from the system.

Overfilling is straightforward. All one has to do is keep filling the vitreous cavity with PFCL. Injecting of PFCL is usually via a double-lumen cannula. One has to withdraw the cannula as one injects the heavy liquid so that the outer sleeve is above the PFCL bubble and in the aqueous. In this way, the PFCL is introduced and the aqueous is removed. The double cannula has to be withdrawn until it is out of the eye (Fig. 4.6). A better way of ensuring total fill is to use a simple single lumen cannula when the eye is nearly filled. This also works so long as there is an open and free flowing port. For example, one can open the three-way tap of the infusion (Fig. 4.7) by simply removing the light pipe and continuing the injection until PFCL flows out of this sclerotomy. It is also useful to tilt the eye slightly so that the draining sclerotomy is uppermost. Overfilling means that the PFCL will fill beyond the anterior edge of the giant retinal tear. There is of course a danger of PFCL going under the retina. In practice, this does not occur, unless there is unrelieved traction. It is not a technique recommended for the giant retinal tear with fixed retinal folds.

With regard to the elimination of all aqueous from the system, filling the eye completely is not difficult. There are no complicated maneuvers and there is no need to visualize the anterior recesses of the eyeball. The only tricky part is maintaining a complete fill. It is often not appreciated that there is a continuous infusion of aqueous. The infusion is used to provide a constant intraocular pressure. As soon as the cannula for injection of PFCL is taken out of the eye, the infusion will run and introduce aqueous back into the eye (Fig. 4.8). Some of the PFCL will be washed out. The total fill is no longer present and the doughnut of aqueous will be re-introduced into the eye!

Even if one takes the precaution to switch over to air after filling the eye totally with PFCL, this is not sufficient. There is aqueous in the infusion line. It is important to fill the infusion line as shown in Fig. 4.7. Otherwise, as soon as an air pump is switched on, this column of aqueous in the infusion line will displace the PFCL and re-establish the doughnut of fluid inside the vitreous cavity as depicted in Fig. 4.8.

It is therefore not sufficient to fill the eye completely; it is necessary to eliminate all aqueous from the system. This means that when the eye is nearly full, the infusion should be disconnected. The PFCL injection should be continued until PFCL fills the infusion tubing as far as the three-way tap to ensure all aqueous is eliminated. For this reason, we have chosen to describe the procedure as "overfilling."

4.5 Injection of Silicone Oil

Once all the aqueous has been eliminated from the vitreous cavity and from the infusion tubing, the priority is to maintain a steady intraocular pressure. There are two ways of achieving this. One is to do a direct silicone oil/PFCL exchange. The other is to perform an air/PFCL exchange then to inject the silicone oil under a constant air infusion.

The first way is probably the easiest. If the infusion cannula is designed for silicone oil injection, then the oil infusion pump can be connected to it and switched on.

It is important to use the appropriate cannula for silicone oil injection. This is particularly the case when highly viscous silicone oil, e.g., 5,700 centistokes oil, is used. Otherwise, the tubing can expand and become disconnected at the points of connection to the metal cannula. Cannulae designed for the injection of silicone oil are usually short with a wide lumen and a strong union between the plastic tubing and the metal cannula. Some surgeons purposely disconnect the normal infusion tubing from the cannula and connect the oil pump via a short length of tubing already filled with silicone oil. Either way, the important point is to avoid prolonged periods of hypotony and re-establish the infusion as soon as possible via the silicone oil pump.

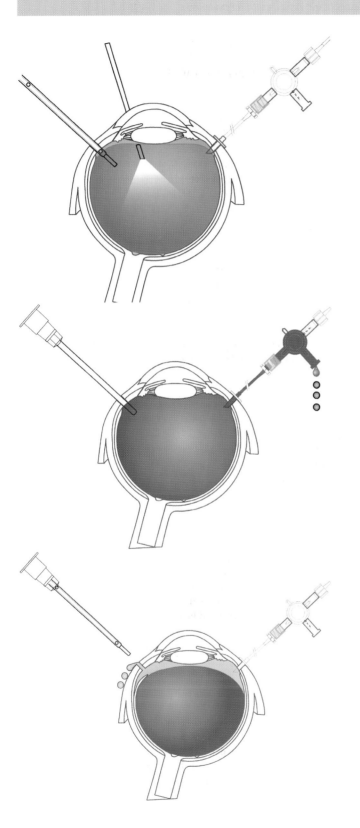

Fig. 4.6 Perfluorocarbon liquids (PFCL) being injected via a double bore cannula

Fig. 4.7 Perfluorocarbon liquids (PFCL) being injected with a single bore cannula; the three-way tap is switched off to the infusion fluid and opened to air. We advocate an overfill, to ensure that all the aqueous is displaced from the system including infusion lines

Fig. 4.8 If the infusion is left running, aqueous can run back in and occupy the space above and around the dome-shaped PFCL bubble. This will encourage slippage

4

The alternative method is equally straightforward. There should be no aqueous in the system, up to and including the three-way tap. The air infusion connected to the three-way tap is then switched on and a normal air/PFCL exchange is then performed. There are no special precautions needed to eliminate any aqueous, as there should be none in the system!

Summary for the Clinician

- Overfilling avoids the need for complicated visualization and manipulation to eliminate the doughnut of fluid.
- It is important to switch off the infusion to avoid the re-introduction of aqueous into the vitreous cavity.
- Overfilling involves the injection of PFCL until all the aqueous is displaced not only from the eye, but also from the infusion tubing including the three-way tap.
- Hypotony should be avoided by connecting the eye to either an oil pump or continuous air infusion.

Acknowledgements

I wish to thank Dr Mariam Ishmail for her work on the NMR images and to Mr Carl Groenewald for his help with the illustrations.

References

1. Wong D, Lois N. Foveal relocation by redistribution of the neurosensory retina. Br J Ophthalmol 2000;84(4):352–357.
2. Wong D, Stanga P, Briggs M, Lenfestey P, Lancaster E, Li KK, et al. Case selection in macular relocation surgery for age related macular degeneration. Br J Ophthalmol 2004;88(2):186–190.
3. Tseng JJ, Barile GR, Schiff WM, Akar Y, Vidne-Hay O, Chang S. Influence of relaxing retinotomy on surgical outcomes in proliferative vitreoretinopathy. Am J Ophthalmol 2005;140(4):628–636.
4. Blumenkranz MS, Azen SP, Aaberg T, Boone DC, Lewis H, Radtke N, et al. Relaxing retinotomy with silicone oil or long-acting gas in eyes with severe proliferative vitreoretinopathy. Silicone Study Report 5. The Silicone Study Group. Am J Ophthalmol 1993;116(5):557–564.
5. Wong D, Williams RL, German MJ. Exchange of perfluorodecalin for gas or oil: a model for avoiding slippage. Graefes Arch Clin Exp Ophthalmol 1998;236(3):234–237.
6. Fawcett IM, Williams RL, Wong D. Contact angles of substances used for internal tamponade in retinal detachment surgery. Graefes Arch Clin Exp Ophthalmol 1994;232(7):438–444.
7. Wong D, Lois N. Perfluorocarbons and semifluorinated alkanes. Semin Ophthalmol 2000;15(1):25–35.
8. Wetterqvist C, Wong D, Williams R, Stappler T, Herbert E, Freeburn S. Tamponade efficiency of perfluorohexyloctane and silicone oil solutions in a model eye chamber. Br J Ophthalmol 2004;88(5):692–696.
9. Wong D, Williams R, Stappler T, Groenewald C. What pressure is exerted on the retina by heavy tamponade agents? Graefes Arch Clin Exp Ophthalmol 2005;243(5):474–477.
10. Chignell AH, Wong D. Management of vitreoretinal disease: a surgical approach. Springer, London, 1998.
11. De Juan E Jr, Loewenstein A, Bressler NM, Alexander J. Translocation of the retina for management of subfoveal choroidal neovascularization. II. A preliminary report in humans. Am J Ophthalmol 1998;125(5):635–646.
12. Lewis H. Macular translocation with chorioscleral outfolding: a pilot clinical study. Am J Ophthalmol 2001;132(2):156–163.
13. De Juan E Jr, Vander JF. Effective macular translocation without scleral imbrication. Am J Ophthalmol 1999;128(3):380–382.
14. Larrison WI, Frederick AR Jr, Peterson TJ, et al. Posterior retinal folds following vitreoretinal surgery. Arch Ophthalmol 1993;111:621–625.
15. Van Meurs JC, Humalda D, Mertens DA, et al. Retinal folds through the macula. Doc Ophthalmol 1991;78:335–340.
16. Pavan PR. Retinal fold in macula following intraocular gas. Arch Ophthalmol 1984;102:83–84.

17. Hayashi A, Usui S, Kawaguchi K, et al. Retinal changes after retinal translocation surgery with scleral imbrication in dog eyes. Invest Ophthalmol Vis Sci 2000;41:4288–4292.

18. Herbert E, Groenewald C, Wong D. Treatment of retinal folds using a modified macula relocation technique with perfluoro-hexyloctane tamponade. Br J Ophthalmol 2003;87(7):921–922.

19. Chang S, Lincoff H, Zimmerman NJ, Fuchs W. Giant retinal tears. Surgical techniques and results using perfluorocarbon liquids. Arch Ophthalmol 1989;107(5):761–766.

20. Han DP, Rychwalski PJ, Mieler WF, Abrams GW. Management of complex retinal detachment with combined relaxing retinotomy and intravitreal perfluoro-n-octane injection. Am J Ophthalmol 1994;118(1):24–32.

21. Erect Indirect Binocular Operating System (Möller Wedel, Haag-Streit group)

22. Spitznas M. A binocular indirect ophthalmomicroscope (BIOM) for non-contact wide-angle vitreous surgery. Graefes Arch Clin Exp Ophthalmol 1987;225(1):13–15.

23. Mathis A, Pagot V, Gazagne C, Malecaze F. Giant retinal tears. Surgical techniques and results using perfluorodecalin and silicone oil tamponade. Retina 1992;12 [3 Suppl]:S7–S10.

Chapter 5

Complete and Early Vitrectomy for Endophthalmitis (CEVE) as Today's Alternative to the Endophthalmitis Vitrectomy Study

5

Ferenc Kuhn, Giampaolo Gini

Core Messages

- Clinical signs of the disease are sufficient to recognize the condition as endophthalmitis and initiate treatment.
- If the attending ophthalmologist does not have the expertise or equipment and thus cannot offer the optimal treatment option, the patient should immediately be referred to a specialist who is able and willing to perform the most promising therapy.
- It is unacceptable to simply inject intravitreal antibiotics and then claim that everything that possibly could have been done has been done to save your eye, but unfortunately the disease has proven to be too tough to conquer.
- The cell wall of the organism may be toxic, and the bacterium may secrete endo- and exotoxins as well as harmful enzymes. This volatile mixture is rather heavy and tends to "sink" toward the deepest point of the vitreous cavity – the macula.

- Early surgical intervention is advantageous since it allows immediate treatment of all treatable pathologies, it serves as a prophylactic measure, preventing complications that would occur with a prolonged disease process, and it reduces the risk of surgery via improved visibility and decreased tissue fragility.
- An overriding principle of surgery is its step-by-step progression from the corneal epithelium toward the macular surface.
- The authors place the pars plana infusion cannula at the beginning of surgery, but do not open the infusion until the position of the cannula can be verified later during the operation.
- If there is a fibrinous membrane that covers the angle, iris, and the anterior surface of the (intraocular) lens, it is crucial not to leave it behind as the membrane can not only hinder visualization, but lead to postoperative intraocular pressure elevation by blocking the angle.
- Early filling of the anterior chamber with viscoelastics has several advantages.
- The intraocular lens is usually left in place.

5

Core Messages

- A large capsulectomy with the vitrectomy probe is always necessary to allow the intravitreal infusion fluid to irrigate the capsular bag; it also improves visualization.
- Unfortunately, even preoperative ultrasonography can be of limited value, or can even be misleading with regard to whether the retina is detached or not.
- The posterior vitreous should be detached and removed over retina that is not necrotic.
- Detachment of the hyaloid anterior to the equator should not be aggressively pursued as this increases the risk of iatrogenic retinal tear formation.
- The risk of permanent visual impairment is almost always smaller from a retinal break than from infection-related retinal destruction.

- The authors strongly believe that the primary line of treatment for the vast majority of eyes with endophthalmitis should be vitrectomy, i.e., purely medical treatment is the exception, not the rule.
- It is not a goal to routinely use silicone oil in the management of endophthalmitis; rather, it represents an exception that is reserved for the worst or most difficult cases. Nevertheless, silicone oil has several unique advantages: it does not allow organism growth, it keeps the retina attached, and it maintains clear media, allowing retinal inspection.
- Statistically significantly better anatomical and functional results are achieved with "complete and early vitrectomy" than in either management arm in the Endophthalmitis Vitrectomy Study.

5.1 Introduction and Definitions

5.1.1 Introduction

Endophthalmitis is a severe, purulent intraocular inflammation. Without proper and timely treatment, the infection results in loss of vision, and commonly in the loss of the eye. It is a clinical entity [3]: even if culturing is unsuccessful in identifying the pathogen, the clinical signs of the disease are sufficient to recognize the condition as endophthalmitis and initiate treatment to fight the infection and its consequences.

Regardless of the etiology, both the organism and the inflammatory response it invokes from the body are harmful to the internal structures of the eye. It is therefore necessary to:

- Recognize the condition early;
- Immediately inform the patient about the condition's characteristics, the therapeutic options, and the prognosis;
- Decide, with the patient's consent [11], on the type of therapy to pursue;
- Execute this therapy in the optimal fashion.

It is also important to remove the ophthalmologist's own ego from the treatment process ("I'm able to handle this situation, I don't need to refer the patient to a colleague") and resist the subconscious reflex to "hide" the patient by relegating him to a remote area of the ward or by sending him home early. If the attending ophthalmologist does not have the expertise or equipment and thus cannot offer the optimal treatment option, the patient should be referred to a specialist who is able and willing to perform the most promising therapy. It is equally unacceptable to simply inject intravitreal antibiotics and then claim that "everything that possibly could have been done has been done to save your eye, but unfortunately the disease has proven to be too tough to conquer."

5.1.2 Definitions

Defining all applicable terms establishes unequivocal communication among opththalmologists, regardless of the individual's place of training or practice. Clarifying certain endophthalmitis-related concepts helps understand the rationale for treatment selection. The definitions and concepts are summarized in Table 5.1.

Table 5.1 Terms and their definitions in the management of endophthalmitis

Term	Definition	Comment
Endophthalmitis	An abscess: intracavital accumulation of purulent material	The eyewall[b] acts like a barrier, a capsule, to effectively shield the purulent process from the rest of the body; this is advantageous because it usually prevents the infection from spreading and thus causing septicemia, but it also concentrates the organism's harmful effects on the tissue it continually bathes: the retina
Early endophthalmitis[a]	An infection with relatively well preserved media clarity, allowing good red reflex, occasionally even observing retinal details	In most cases,[c] the initial signs of endophthalmitis are discrete[d] and the progression is relatively slow. This, however, should not make the ophthalmologist complacent: the infecting organism is rarely known at this point, and the process can rapidly turn for the worst. This is why it is misleading to term an early endophthalmitis "mild"
Advanced endophthalmitis[a]	An infection with severe opacity in the anterior media, typically accompanied by severe vitreous infiltration or true abscess	An (almost) end stage condition, where functional failure is certain and anatomical failure is likely
Anatomical failure[a]	Enucleation, evisceration, or phthisis	The ophthalmologist is either forced to enucleate/eviscerate the eye to cure the infection and prevent its spread, or the infection, even if cured, eventually shuts down aqueous production and the eye becomes phthisical – which can later lead to enucleation or evisceration for cosmetical reasons
Endophthalmitis maculopathy[a]	Macular injury (edema, stress hemorrhage, epimacular proliferation) as a result of the infection	These consequences may result from the organism or the inflammatory reaction of the body; they can cause permanent (i.e., unimproveable) damage or one that requires additional medical therapy or surgery. Even if the therapy results in anatomical success, the functional recovery may not be complete
Macular hypopyon[a]	Accumulation of purulent material in the macular area	The purulent material is heavier than the vitreous/fluid; as most patients spend most of their time in the supine position, the material settles on the lowest point of the eye, typically causing disproportionally more severe damage here

[a]Modified after Morris and Witherspoon who originally introduced the concept [11]

[b]Cornea and sclera

[c]An obvious exception is an infection caused by *Bacillus* sp.

[d]Especially if the infection is restricted to the anterior chamber and the anterior vitreous

5.2 Etiology and Classification

The pathogen may be exogenous or endogenous. Of the former, we distinguish between those caused by trauma or surgery; the latter may follow trabeculectomy or other types of surgery (most commonly cataract extraction). Such postoperative endophthalmitis may be acute (presenting within a few weeks of surgery) or chronic. (This chapter was written on the management of eyes with the same inclusion criteria as those in the Endophthalmitis Vitrectomy Study (EVS): acute postoperative endophthalmitis occurring within 6 weeks of cataract extraction with intraocular lens implantation or of secondary intraocular lens implantation. Treating eyes with endophthalmitis of other etiologies or chronicity requires a somewhat modified strategy, including timing and surgical details. These are not discussed here.)

5.3 Pathophysiology, Organisms, and Diagnostics in Brief

5.3.1 Pathophysiology

The intravitreal organism causes severe inflammation – indeed, some of the most significant visual consequences of the infection, such as cystoid macular edema and epimacular membrane formation, are caused by the body's response, rather than by the organism directly. In addition, the cell wall of the organism may be toxic, and the bacterium may secrete endo- and exotoxins as well as harmful enzymes. These lead to various retinal pathologies, including widespread necrosis. This volatile mixture (inflammatory debris, including organism, white blood cells, humoral agents, etc.) is rather heavy and tends to "sink" toward the deepest point of the vitreous cavity.

5.3.2 Organisms

Table 5.2 lists the most commonly encountered organisms in acute postoperative endophthalmitis. Virulence of the pathogen for the clinician is indicated by how early after surgery the infection presents, how rapidly the disease progresses from early to advanced, and how severe the signs are.

5.3.3 Diagnostics

5.3.3.1 Clinical

Most or all of the following signs/symptoms are present:
- Pain;
- Red ("hot"), inflamed eye, dilated conjunctival and ciliary blood vessels;
- Reduced corneal clarity due to edema;
- Hazy anterior chamber due to fibrin, cells, bacteria, increased protein content, occasionally blood; hypopyon is usually also found (a hypopyon may become invisible simply because the patient is in bed);

Table 5.2 The most common organisms in acute postoperative endophthalmitis[a]

Organism	Comment
Staphylococcus epidermidis	Relatively nonvirulent; by far the most common organism (40–70%), especially in diabetics
Staphylococcus aureus	Quite virulent; 10–20% of those with positive culture
Streptococcus species	Quite virulent; 6–9% of those with positive culture
Gram-negative rods (Proteus, Pseudomonas, Serratia)	Virulent; relatively rare
Bacillus species	Very virulent; extremely rare

[a]Based on an extensive literature survey

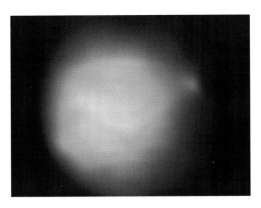

Fig. 5.1 Macular hypopyon. Intraoperative image: accumulation of purulent material over the macula in a patient with postoperative endophthalmitis

- Formation of a fibrinous membrane over the crystalline/intraocular lens and the iris;
- Constricted pupil (which may be masked by dilating drugs prescribed postoperatively);
- Reduced or nonexistent red reflex;
- Vitreous opacity of varying degrees, with foci of pus or abscess/es;
- If the retina can be visualized, endophthalmitis retinopathy: stress hemorrhages, sheathed vessels, necrotic areas, macular swelling, macular hypopyon (Fig. 5.1).

5.3.3.2 Other

Typical appearance on ultrasonography; culture from the anterior chamber and vitreous. These are not discussed in this chapter.

5.4 Principles of Therapy

The intervention aims to:
- Kill the organism;
- Remove the inflammatory debris from the vitreous cavity;
- Block the inflammatory cascade and its effects on the retina;
- Treat the complications of the infection;
- Minimize future complications, whether from the infection or from the treatment itself;

- Intervene as soon as possible. Endophthalmitis is an emergency and must be treated as one. Timing of the intervention is where the surgeon's error (i.e., delay in initiating proper treatment) is most easily controllable.

Summary for the Clinician:

■ Without proper and timely treatment, the infection results in loss of vision, and commonly in the loss of the eye.
■ The cell wall of the organism may be toxic, and the bacterium may secrete endo- and exotoxins as well as harmful enzymes. These lead to various retinal pathologies, including widespread necrosis.
■ Some of the most significant visual consequences of the infection, such as cystoid macular edema and epimacular membrane formation, are caused by the body's response, rather than by the organism directly.
■ Virulence of the pathogen for the clinician is indicated by how early after surgery the infection presents, how rapidly the disease progresses from early to advanced, and how severe the signs are.
■ The most important signs/symptoms of endophthalmitis are: pain, haze, hypopyon, and endophthalmitis retinopathy.
■ Principles of therapy are: killing the organism, removing the inflammatory debris, and to intervene as soon as possible.

5.5 The EVS

5.5.1 Study Design

Conducted between January 1990 and January 1994, the EVS [4] was a prospective, randomized, multicenter trial on 420 eyes to determine whether it is necessary in acute postoperative endophthalmitis to use systemic antibiotics or perform routine immediate vitrectomy (Table 5.3).

Table 5.3 Design of the Endophthalmitis Vitrectomy Study (EVS)

	Vitrectomy	No vitrectomy
Intravenous antibiotics	106[a]	100[a]
No intravenous antibiotics	112[a]	102[a]

[a]Number of eyes in each group; total: 420 eyes

5.5.2 Results

Statistical analysis of the EVS findings led the study authors to the following conclusions:

- Systemic antibiotics do not improve the outcome;
- Vitrectomy is indicated only in eyes with light perception vision.

5.5.3 Consequences of the EVS Recommendations

Vitrectomy for endophthalmitis was becoming increasingly popular [3] when the publication of the EVS in 1995 dramatically and abruptly changed the treatment philosophy. As advocated by the EVS, vitrectomy is now reserved for the most severe cases, and this vitrectomy is limited to the anterior vitreous. (Systemic antibiotics are still used by many ophthalmologists.) The following quote is a typical example: "If a vitrectomy is indicated (e.g., a patient with visual acuity of light perception…), a core vitrectomy should be performed, and no attempt should be made to excise the cortical…vitreous" [6]. This management approach is now typical even in countries where the ophthalmologist's decisions can still be made based on purely medical, rather than on medicolegal or insurance company-forced reasoning.

5.6 Rationale for Performing Complete and Early Vitrectomy for Endophthalmitis

The following presents a systematic, logic- and experience-based (re)consideration of the advantages of a surgical approach to eyes with endophthalmitis [7].

5.6.1 Why Perform Vitrectomy?

Surgery has several advantages over conservative therapy. Vitrectomy:

- Increases retinal oxygenization [13];
- Provides a large specimen for diagnostic evaluation;
- Allows definite treatment at a time when the organism (and its virulence) is still unknown (i.e., antibiotic selection is based on statistical probability, not on case-specific information);
- Dramatically reduces the inflammatory debris load in the vitreous cavity, thereby lessening its harmful effect on the retina and other intraocular tissues;
- Reduces the incidence and severity of macular complications;
- Allows direct inspection of the retina by removing the nontransparent medium, thereby permitting timely treatment of coexisting or developing pathologies;
- Increases the access to the retina of intravitreally administered pharmacological agents;
- Reduces the duration of the disease, thus accelerating visual rehabilitation;
- Reduces the incidence and severity of retinal, especially macular, complications.

5.6.2 Why Perform Early Vitrectomy?

As mentioned earlier, endophthalmitis is a process that progressively destroys the intraocular tissues it bathes. Early surgical intervention is advantageous since it:

- Allows immediate treatment of all treatable pathologies;
- Serves as a prophylactic measure, preventing complications that would occur with a prolonged disease process;

- Reduces the risk of surgery via improved visibility (as the disease progresses, the corneal transparency decreases due to increasing edema) and decreased tissue fragility (the less severe the existing pathology, the less likely that iatrogenic complications will occur).

5.6.3 Why Perform Complete Vitrectomy?

The inflammatory debris, as mentioned earlier, is heavy, and typically settles over the posterior pole since most patients spend most of their days lying in bed.

If vitrectomy is not complete (see the instructions in the "Methods" section of the EVS ["If there was no posterior vitreous separation, no attempt was made to induce a vitreous detachment, and the posterior cortical vitreous was not aggressively removed. It was a goal of surgery to remove at least 50% of the vitreous gel in eyes with no vitreous separation."] [4]), the part that is not removed is obviously the posterior half. Only by detaching the posterior hyaloid does the surgeon gain access to the "naked" retinal surface, allowing complete removal of the pus and debris that have accumulated there (macular hypopyon). (Contrary to popular belief, the posterior vitreous cortex remains attached to the retina in the majority of cases. What appears in many eyes as vitreous detachment is often vitreoschisis; no current preoperative evaluation method allows absolute determination with regard to whether a posterior vitreous detachment exists). Complete vitrectomy, however, implies detachment and removal of the vitreous posteriorly, not in the periphery, where the surgeon must be more conservative (see below).

- Conclusions from the EVS: systemic antibiotics do not improve the outcome; vitrectomy is indicated only in eyes with light perception vision.
- Consequences of the EVS: if a vitrectomy is indicated a core vitrectomy should be performed, and no attempt should be made to excise the cortical vitreous.
- Complete and early vitrectomy for endophthalmitis, on the other hand, dramatically reduces the inflammatory debris load in the

vitreous cavity and provides a large specimen for diagnostic evaluation.
- Complete and early vitrectomy for endophthalmitis allows definite treatment, reduces the incidence and severity of retinal, especially macular, complications. Early vitrectomy reduces the risk of surgery via improved visibility and decreased tissue fragility.
- Only a complete vitrectomy allows detachment of the posterior hyaloid and complete removal of the pus and debris.

5.7 Complete and Early Vitrectomy for Endophthalmitis: Surgical Steps

Cases in which the eye is still phakic are included. It must be emphasized that what is described here presents the desired, optimal case. The surgeon must be ready to accept compromises if visibility is too poor to allow fine intravitreal maneuvers or if the retina is too necrotic to permit manipulations such as posterior vitreous detachment. An overriding principle of surgery is its step-by-step progression from the corneal epithelium toward the macular surface. No step described here should be skipped as this may result in surgical compromises that may not otherwise have been necessary and that can impair the functional outcome.

The benefits of a wide-angle viewing system cannot be overemphasized. It makes otherwise difficult surgery much easier to perform, and dramatically increases safety and efficacy.

5.7.1 Initial Steps

Prepare the eye as for any intraocular surgery; be especially careful if the fellow eye had surgery recently. Make sure that if no "septic" operating room is available for the surgery, a proper protocol is in place to clean/sterilize the operating room afterward. The authors perform most of their surgery under local anesthesia. Prepare your diagnostic kit in time so that culturing is efficient in terms of sterility, media availability, delivery to the lab, and processing in the lab. Make sure that no undue pressure is exerted on the eye when

5

placing the lid speculum (or retracting sutures if necessary): the eye is "hot" and the intraocular pressure may be high, therefore the risk of intra-operative hemorrhage [8] is not negligible. The authors place the pars plana infusion cannula at the beginning of surgery, but do not open the infusion until the cannula's position can be verified later during the operation. (The initial tool for providing intraocular infusion is typically an anterior chamber maintainer.)

5.7.2 Cornea

As the epithelium is always edematous, its removal is necessary in virtually every case, even in diabetics. Scraping the epithelium dramatically increases visibility of the deeper structures and thus increases the safety and scope of surgery. Do not remove the epithelium in the limbus (removing the stem cells interferes with re-epithelialization) and be careful not to damage Bowman's membrane. If the stroma also has significant edema, the surgeon may try to press a dry sponge against it, or use topical high-concentration glucose. It is uncommon, though, for stromal edema to significantly impair visibility. Descemet's folds may also be a problem, see below. If visibility through the cornea remains compromised despite all efforts, there are several options:

- Vitrectomy may be delayed until topical corticosteroids are successful in improving media clarity. This must be weighed against the damage inflicted by the ongoing disease process.
- Vitrectomy may be performed in a limited fashion, consistent with safety [10]. ("proportional pars plana vitrectomy" [PPPV], a term coined by R. Morris [10]). This must be weighed against the damage inflicted by the ongoing disease process.
- An endoscope may be utilized [2]. This requires not only availability of the equipment, but also considerable experience on the surgeon's part.
- A temporary keratoprosthesis (TKP) can be placed [12], followed by implantation of a donor cornea at the conclusion of surgery (Fig. 5.2). If no donor cornea is available, even the original corneal button may be temporarily reused. Use of a TKP requires availability

of the device and expertise in its use as well as extensive knowledge of postoperative handling of the transplant.

5.7.3 Anterior Chamber

There are several instruments/techniques to rid the anterior chamber of *loose debris*: with an irrigation–aspiration cannula; via irrigation and then aspiration through a single paracentesis; using an anterior chamber maintainer while aspirating through a separate paracentesis, etc. The vitrectomy probe is usually preferred by the authors since this also allows cutting if some formidable material is engaged. It is mandatory to always have some type of irrigation in place before aspirating, even if the material to be removed is apparently of insignificant volume: collapse of the anterior chamber – a sudden drop in the intraocular pressure – risks severe hemorrhage. The angle is typically also full of debris and should be thoroughly irrigated. The material ultimately removed is usually much more voluminous than presumed.

There is almost always a fibrinous membrane that covers the angle, iris, and the anterior surface of the (intraocular) lens. The membrane may be relatively thin, barely visible until engaged,

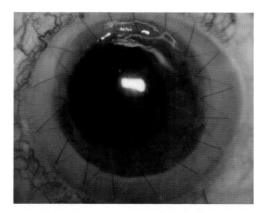

Fig. 5.2 Corneal transplantation after complete and early vitrectomy for endophthalmitis (CEVE). Five weeks afterward, a temporary keratoprosthesis (TKP) was necessary to allow treatment of endophthalmitis with severe retinal complications. The corneal graft is clear with no signs of rejection

but can also be fairly substantial. It is rather elastic and very sticky (adhesion) – but also strong (cohesion). Once grabbed by a vacuum (cannula, vitrectomy probe) or forceps, it is usually possible to remove it in its entirety and in one piece. It is crucial not to leave it behind as the membrane can not only hinder visualization, but lead to postoperative intraocular pressure elevation by blocking the angle. The membrane occasionally reoccurs during surgery, especially in children, requiring repeat removal.

Early filling of the anterior chamber with viscoelastics has several advantages. It:

- Prevents reaccumulation of the inflammatory debris;
- Reduces the risk of bleeding;
- Pushes/keeps out of the visual axis any fresh blood or other debris;
- Keeps the anterior chamber formed;
- Keeps the pupil dilated;
- Reduces Descemet's folds.

5.7.4 Pupil

A large pupillary opening greatly enhances visibility of the posterior segment. If dilating agents – including intracameral adrenalin – are insufficient and neither do viscoelastics help, iris retractors should be used.

5.7.5 (Intraocular) Lens

The crystalline lens is usually left in place. If its anterior surface is "dirty" and cannot be displaced with viscoelastics, and it impairs posterior segment manipulations, the lens should be sacrificed. Whether lensectomy or phacoemulsification is performed is an individual decision. (It is the surgeon's decision as to whether any of the lens capsules is retained; the focus should be on saving the eye, not "the bag for optimal subsequent placement of an intraocular lens.") The rule is: saving the lens or any of its capsules should not compromise curing the infection or its consequences.

The intraocular lens is usually left in place. If its anterior surface is "dirty" it should be wiped clean with a sponge, a small piece of cotton held in intravitreal forceps, or some other tool (for instance, a Tano membrane scraper).

5.7.6 Posterior Lens Capsule

A large capsulectomy with the vitrectomy probe is always necessary to allow the intravitreal infusion fluid to irrigate the capsular bag (irrigation through the pars plana/posterior capsulectomy with antibiotic solution using a syringe may also have to be performed); it also improves visualization. (The bag, and the intraocular lens, must be removed if the endophthalmitis is chronic.) Occasionally, the posterior surface of the intraocular lens must also be wiped clean.

5.7.7 Vitrectomy

There is a considerable future for 23- and even 25-gauge systems; however, a smaller gauge and the lack of having to suture the sclerotomies is no justification for incomplete vitreous removal. The sequence of vitreous removal is primarily determined by the clarity of the vitreous. A relatively transparent vitreous allows posterio-anterior vitrectomy [9], which the authors prefer: the posterior vitreous is detached first, followed by vitreous removal that is progressively anterior in its direction. If the vitreous is moderately hazy, removal should start behind the lens and advance carefully, slowly, toward the retina. Once the posterior pole is reached and the hyaloid is detached there, vitrectomy is completed by moving the probe anteriorly. If the vitreous is very hazy, surgery becomes extremely difficult. There are several vitreous layers present, which are shaped (like onion peel). There may be streaks of blood among the layers, giving the appearance of a detached retina; conversely, the retina may be necrotic and not bleed when cut into. (Such a condition represents one of the most challenging indications for vitrectomy. Even for experienced surgeons, distinguishing between white vitreous layers with streaks of hemorrhage and a white, necrotic retina without patent blood vessels may be extremely difficult.) A less experienced or careful surgeon may remove large chunks of the retina before realizing what he has "bitten into."

5

Unfortunately, even preoperative ultrasonography can be of no value, or even be misleading, with regard to whether or not the retina is detached (Fig. 5.3).

The least risky technique in such eyes is to "dig" a vertical "well" nasally (rather than, as first instinct would suggest, carefully peeling the onion layers by moving the vitrectomy probe in horizontal sweeps); the surgeon may create a small retinal break, but once the vitrectomy probe is behind the retina, the anatomical situation becomes much clearer. It is helpful to use the vitrectomy probe and the flute needle alternately: the latter can vacuum the typical grayish fluid that otherwise blocks the surgeon's view. Once the cleavage plane between vitreous and retina has been found, heavy liquids, among other tools, can be used to separate the retina from the vitreous. Vitreous separation and removal is usually possible even if the retina is already detached (Fig. 5.4).

Unless the vitreous is very hazy, the posterior hyaloid is rather easy to identify since it is somewhat opaque, not transparent as usual. Occa-sionally, colonies of bacteria may be present on it surface (appearing as multiple white [yellowish] dots), also helping identification. If the surgeon is in doubt, a single drop of filtered triamcinolone helps identify it. The hyaloid is carefully lifted; if the retina is necrotic and would also detach, the vitreous is only trimmed over this area (Fig. 5.5). The posterior vitreous, however, should be detached and removed over retina that is not necrotic. The retinal appearance instantly changes to a clear image once the vitreous "veil" has been lifted. The central vitreous must be completely removed to minimize the bacterial load ("reservoir") inside the eye.

Detachment of the hyaloid anterior to the equator should not be aggressively pursued as this increases the risk of iatrogenic retinal tear formation. Only trimming is recommended in the periphery to reduce the incidence of iatrogenic retinal injury. Careful trimming is sufficient to reduce the volume of the infected medium while keeping the retinal injury risk at an acceptably low level. (In other words: posterior vitreous removal in complete and early vitrec-

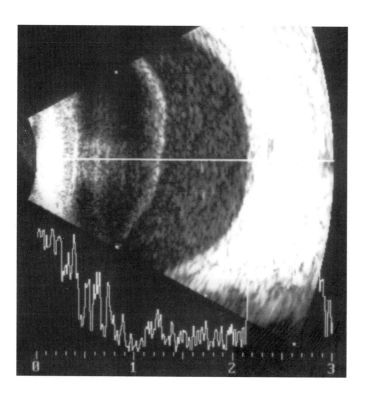

Fig. 5.3 Ultrasound imaging of an eye with hazy vitreous due to endophthalmitis. The preoperative image suggests posterior vitreous detachment with subhyaloid infiltration. During surgery, however, a nondetached vitreous was found with a complete retinal detachment and a subretinal fluid rich in protein and cellular elements

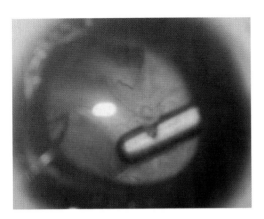

Fig. 5.4 Complete and early vitrectomy for endophthalmitis in an eye with detached retina. If the retina is detached, separation and then removal of the still attached vitreous requires careful manipulation with the vitrectomy probe, occasionally also requiring the use of other tools (see the text for more details)

tomy for endophthalmitis (CEVE) is just the opposite of what the EVS recommended; there is similarity between the CEVE and EVS regarding peripheral vitrectomy.)

5.7.8 When to Stop Vitreous Removal?

This is an important question that only experience can answer in each individual case. The surgeon faces two, antagonistic treatment goals:
- Curing the infection requires as complete a vitrectomy as possible;

- Vitreous removal should be performed without creating iatrogenic retinal damage.

This conflict is not an easy one to resolve. As a general rule, the primary goal is to cure the infection. If a retinal break is created, however, this does not represent a death sentence for the eye (an ongoing infection may be). The risk of permanent visual impairment is almost always smaller from a retinal break than from infection-related retinal destruction. Treatment of a retinal break or detachment is a routine procedure for the vitreoretinal surgeon (see below).

5.7.9 Retina

The macular surface should always be vacuumed, even if there is no apparent pus accumulation on it. The silicone-tipped flute needle is used with passive, not active, suction. Even if larger pus fragments are present, these tend to break up and can easily exit the eye through the needle. Alternatively, the vitrectomy probe's aspiration is utilized once the sticky material has been mobilized from the macular surface. It is rarely necessary to meticulously vacuum the retinal surface elsewhere.

If areas of necrosis are encountered, these may be surrounded by rows of laser treatment, once the vitreous is trimmed/removed. (Laser treatment presumes a healthy retina and pigment epithelium in the adjacent areas.) Other coexisting pathologies (e.g., tears, detachment) are also treated as if appearing in an eye without

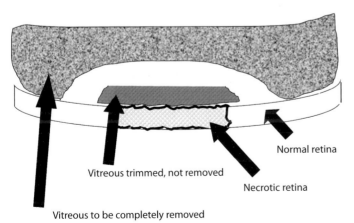

Normal retina

Vitreous trimmed, not removed

Necrotic retina

Vitreous to be completely removed

Fig. 5.5 Trimming the vitreous over necrotic retina. Instead of detaching the posterior hyaloid, it is trimmed parallel to the retina, then cut circumferentially, allowing safe detachment and removal of the vitreous in the adjacent area. (Schematic representation, cross-sectional image)

infection. Gas tamponade may also be used, and medications can be injected into an eye with tamponade. (Alternatively, an incomplete fluid–gas exchange is performed and the drugs are injected into the fluid component.) The use of silicone oil tamponade is discussed separately below.

5.7.10 Enucleation/Evisceration

These are performed only if absolutely necessary: an infection that is (about to be) breaking through the sclera and causing panophthalmitis (tissue melting) or an eye whose anatomy cannot be restored to normal appearance and there is no hope for even light perception vision. Extensive counseling [11] must precede eye removal.

5.7.11 Pharmacological Treatment

It is not the scope of this chapter to discuss this in detail. The authors use heavy topical, occasionally subconjunctival, antibiotic and corticosteroid treatment in every case; antibiotics and corticosteroid intravitreally; and oral antibiotics [5]. (Even if there is corneal erosion; the benefits more than outweigh the risks. Topical corticosteroid therapy, however, is discontinued after 1 week if the erosion remains unhealed.) Intraoperatively, the authors use antibiotics and corticosteroids in the infusion fluid only if silicone oil is to be used (see below).

5.8 Surgical Decision-Making and Complications

5.8.1 Decision-Making

It must be emphasized that the decision whether to undergo surgery is the patient's; the ophthalmologist should inform the patient about the condition and the risks/benefits of each treatment option in a way that allows the patient to make a choice that he is comfortable with [9]. The authors strongly believe that the primary line of treatment for the vast majority of eyes with endophthalmitis should be vitrectomy; i.e., purely medical treatment is the exception, not the rule (Fig. 5.6). The decision whether surgery

is performed is driven not by the visual acuity (i.e., light perception versus better, see the EVS recommendation [3]), but by the clinical appearance and course. This is especially important since deterioration can be rapid, leading to irreversible but otherwise preventable damage.

If performed on an eye with early disease, the risk of serious retinal complications is no greater than it is for other conditions such as a "simple" vitreous hemorrhage. Vitreoretinal surgeons with decent experience should be able to perform this surgery.

With increasingly advanced cases, the degree of surgical difficulties and the risk of complications grow exponentially. It is therefore best for the less experienced surgeon to refer such cases.

Finally, the authors do not automatically render an eye with no light perception vision inoperable [12]. If the eye had good vision before, the loss of light perception is recent, the eye's anatomical condition permits surgery, and the patient understands that the chance of visual improvement is low, surgery should be offered as an option. Cleaning the eye's interior, even if light perception does not return, helps cosmesis, comfort, and reduces the incidence of enucleation/evisceration. (Eye removal is a major additional psychological trauma to the patient.)

5.8.2 Complications and Their Management

Only retinal complications are discussed here; it must also be understood that these can occur as the result of the disease itself, not only as a surgical complication.

5.8.2.1 Retinal Break

Breaks can occur via several mechanisms (e.g., as a "normal" complication in the periphery, as a direct injury from an intravitreal instrument, or as a result of trying to detach the vitreous over a necrotic retina [a common site, not surprisingly, is the fovea.]). The breaks can be surrounded with laser or if longer-term tamponade is felt necessary, silicone oil may be used; the laser treatment can be deferred.

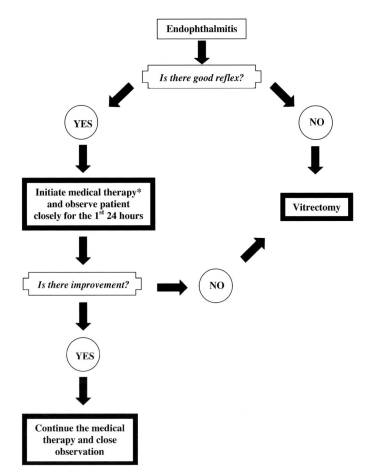

Fig. 5.6 Treatment algorithm of CEVE for acute postoperative endophthalmitis

5.8.2.2 Retinal Detachment

Whether caused by the disease or, less commonly, by the surgeon, a retinal detachment is treated as if occurring in a noninfected eye. First the vitreous (and pus) removal is completed, then the break is sealed with laser (see above) once the subretinal fluid is removed, and some type of tamponade is used. The fact that this is an eye with endophthalmitis should have no bearing on the choice of the tamponade.

5.8.2.3 Silicone Oil as a Long-Term Tamponade

The authors consider using silicone oil if they know they have created a retinal break or are uncertain whether or not they have; if a retinal

detachment is present; or if there are large areas of retinal necrosis.

It is not a goal to routinely use silicone oil in the management of endophthalmitis; rather, it represents an exception, reserved for the worst/most difficult cases. Nevertheless, silicone oil has several unique advantages:
- Bacteria do not multiply in silicone oil [1];
- Silicone oil prevents/treats retinal detachment of a rhegmatogenous nature;
- The intravitreal silicone oil remains clear, allowing visualization of the retina throughout the postoperative period.

A few rules about silicone oil use in eyes with endophthalmitis must be observed:
- Do not implant silicone oil if the vitreous cavity has not been adequately cleansed. The remaining pathogens, while unable to freely

5

circulate, may be pressed against a circumscribed area, causing localized retinal damage.

- The authors use antibiotics and corticosteroids in the infusion fluid if silicone oil is to be used. (Without silicone oil use, medications are not used in the infusion fluid.) The dosages are identical to those used in an intravitreal injection (i.e., the drugs are not diluted).
- Antibiotics and corticosteroids are injected into the oil at the end of the procedure. As demonstrated by the authors, triamcinolone is observed to be spread fairly evenly against the retinal surface the next day. (Appears as a ping-pong ball immediately after the injection.)

5.9 Results with CEVE and Their Comparison with the EVS

Table 5.4 shows the results the authors achieved in a consecutive series of 47 eyes with acute postoperative endophthalmitis. The inclusion criteria were identical to those used in the EVS except that eyes were not excluded, as in the EVS, for lack of iris visibility due to corneal or anterior chamber problems, nor for the presence of even high retinal detachment. (If anything, the cohort in the authors' series was in worse condition than eyes in the EVS.) Although the authors' study was not randomized or prospective, the selection criteria allow a careful comparison between the two studies (Table 5.4).

Statistically significantly better anatomical and functional results were found with CEVE than in either management arm in the EVS. The authors attribute this improvement to vitrectomy being early (in other words: vitrectomy is the primary treatment option; its application is the rule, not the exception) and complete, and to its being the primary line of treatment, rather than being applied as a last resort.

Summary for the Clinician

- An overriding principle of surgery is its step-by-step progression from the corneal epithelium toward the macular surface.
- Make sure that no undue pressure is exerted on the eye.
- Do not open the pars plana infusion until the cannula's position can be verified later during the operation.
- Scraping the epithelium dramatically increases visibility of the deeper structures and thus increases the safety and scope of surgery.
- It is mandatory to always have some type of irrigation in place before aspirating.

Table 5.4 Results with complete and early vitrectomy for endophthalmitis (CEVE) and their comparison with those in the EVS

Variable	EVS, vitrectomy	EVS, no vitrectomy	CEVE
Number of eyes	218	202	47
Retinal detachment*	2.9%	7.2%	0%
Enucleation/evisceration/phthisis*	2.5%	6.2%	0%
Expulsive hemorrhage*	1.9%	4.9%	0%
Repeat vitrectomy*	0%	6.0%	0%
No light perception final vision*	4%	5%	0%
Final visual acuity 20/40 or greater*	54%	52%	91%

*$p<0.0001$, Fisher's exact test, comparing EVS and CEVE outcomes

Summary for the Clinician

- Early filling of the anterior chamber with viscoelastics has several advantages.
- Saving the lens or any of its capsules should not compromise curing the infection or its consequences.
- Unless the vitreous is very hazy, the posterior hyaloid is rather easy to identify since it is somewhat opaque, not transparent as usual. If the vitreous is hazy, however, surgery is very difficult, and considerable experience is required to distinguish between vitreous layers and the necrotic, occasionally already detached retina.
- The central vitreous must be completely removed to minimize the bacterial load ("reservoir") inside the eye.
- Curing the infection requires as complete a vitrectomy as possible; if the vitreous cannot be separated from necrotic retina, it must be circumcised (trimmed), to avoid creating an iatrogenic retinal detachment. This is rare, however, and represents a strong argument in favor of early rather than late intervention.
- The macular surface should always be vacuumed.
- The decision regarding whether or not surgery is performed is driven not by the visual acuity but by the clinical appearance and course.
- With increasingly advanced cases, the degree of surgical difficulties and the risk of complications grow exponentially. It is therefore best for the less experienced surgeon to refer such cases.
- Silicone oil is reserved for the worst/most difficult cases. Bacteria do not multiply in silicone oil. The "dead space" for therapeutic antibiotic levels is eliminated. Intravitreal drug dosages are identical to those used in eyes without vitreous substitutes.

5.10 Summary and Recommendations

The organizers of the EVS deserve a lot of credit for introducing a systematic, statistically well-analyzed approach to the management of eyes with acute postoperative endophthalmitis. Because of the fear of iatrogenic retinal damage during an operation where visibility is a serious problem, however, the EVS protocol called for a vitrectomy that was not radical. Indeed, the EVS compared eyes with no vitrectomy (small, diagnostic biopsy) with eyes with limited vitrectomy (medium biopsy). As a result, the EVS was unable to demonstrate any difference between surgical and nonsurgical treatment, except in eyes that were in their final stage of damage. (It is very likely that if vitrectomy in the surgical arm of the EVS had been complete, similar outcomes would have been found.)

Two decades have passed since planning for the EVS started. Among other factors, better understanding of the pathophysiology, safer vitrectomy machines, improved intraoperative visualization technologies, increasingly efficacious techniques of retinal reattachment (now there is fear of the infection more than of the complications of surgery), new antibiotics (more effective/potent and able to penetrate the blood–retina barrier in higher concentrations) are now available; consequently, it is time to reevaluate the role of vitrectomy in the treatment of eyes with acute postoperative endophthalmitis.

If we compare the "no-vitrectomy" and "partial" vitrectomy arms of the EVS, we must notice that the surgical group faired better in terms of retinal detachment, anatomical failure, expulsive hemorrhage, and reoperation rates. If we compare these results with those achieved with CEVE, both the anatomical and functional outcomes show a statistically significant improvement over either of the EVS groups. The authors therefore strongly advocate the CEVE approach, and also recommend using new generation systemic antibiotics: administered orally, these reach the vitreous cavity in sufficiently high concentration, providing for "bacterial kill"; removal of the inflammatory debris then completes the process, allowing maximum treatment of an otherwise sight-threatening condition.

5

A.C. Celsus declared two millennia ago: "*Ubi pus, ibi evacua*." Today, when vitrectomy is a routine procedure and our armamentarium to treat not only an ever-growing array of conditions, but also the occasional complications of surgery, CEVE for acute postoperative endophthalmitis is proving to be a superior approach than recommended by the EVS in 1995.

References

1.   Aras C, Ozdamar A, Karacorlu M, Ozkan S (2002) Silicone oil in the surgical treatment of endophthalmitis associated with retinal detachment. Int Ophthalmol 24:147–150
2.   Boscher C, Amar R, Lebuisson DA (2002) Endoscopy assisted vitrectomy (EAV) for severe endophthalmitis with visual acuity limited to light perception. Joint Retina and Vitreous Societies meeting, San Francisco, CA, September 2002.
3.   Chen CJ (1983) Management of infectious endophthalmitis by combined vitrectomy and intraocular injection. Ann Ophthalmol 15:968–979
4.   Endophthalmitis Vitrectomy Study Group (1995) Results of the Endophthalmitis Vitrectomy Study. Arch Ophthalmol 113:1479–1496
5.   Hariprasad SM, Shah GK, Mieler WF, Feiner L, Blinder KJ, Holekamp NM, Gao H, Prince RA (2006) Vitreous and aqueous penetration of orally administered moxifloxacin in humans. Arch Ophthalmol 124:178–182
6.   Kresloff M, Castellarin A, Zarbin M (1998) Endophthalmitis. Surv Ophthalmol 43:193–224.
7.   Kuhn F, Gini G (2005) Ten years after…are findings of the Endophthalmitis Vitrectomy Study still relevant today? Graefes Arch Clin Exp Ophthalmol 243:1197–1199
8.   Kuhn F, Morris R, Mester V, Witherspoon CD (1998) Management of intraoperative expulsive choroidal hemorrhage during anterior segment surgery. In: Stirpe M (ed) Anterior and posterior segment surgery: mutual problems and common interests. Ophthalmic Communications Society, New York, pp 191–203
9.   Kuhn F, Kiss Gy, Mester V, Szijarto Zs, Kovacs B (2004) Vitrectomy with internal limiting membrane removal for clinically significant macular edema. Graefes Arch Clin Exp Ophthalmol 242:402–408
10. Morris R, Witherspoon CD, Kuhn F, Bryne JB, Endophthalmitis. In: Roy FH (1995) Masters techniques in ophthalmology. Williams and Wilkins, pp 560–572
11. Morris R, Kuhn F, Witherspoon CD (1998) Counseling the eye trauma victim. In: Alfaro V, Liggett P (eds) Vitrectomy in the management of the injured globe. Lippincott Raven, Philadelphia, pp 25–29
12. Morris R, Kuhn F, Witherspoon CD (1998) Management of the recently injured eye with no light perception vision. In: Alfaro V, Liggett P (eds) Vitrectomy in the management of the injured globe. Lippincott Raven, Philadelphia, pp 113–125
13. Stefansson E, Novack RL, Hatchell DL (1990) Vitrectomy prevents retinal hypoxia in branch retinal vein occlusion. Invest Ophthalmol Vis Sc 31:284–289

Treatment of Acute Bacterial Endophthalmitis After Cataract Surgery Without Vitrectomy

6

Thomas Theelen, Maurits A.D. Tilanus

Core Messages

- Exogenous endophthalmitis due to cataract surgery is rare and occurs in approximately 0.05% of all cases with a growing incidence since the routine use of no-stitch cataract surgery began.
- Most of the patients with acute endophthalmitis after cataract surgery become symptomatic between 1 day and 2 weeks after surgery.
- When the diagnosis endophthalmitis has been made a medical emergency is present and the next diagnostic and therapeutic steps do not permit any delays. We strongly advise carrying out a vitreous tap and injecting antibiotics into the vitreous cavity within less than an hour after the clinical diagnosis.
- Vitreoretinal specialists all over the world are divided into two camps: those who avoid early vitrectomy and those who claim the obligation of immediate complete pars plana vitrectomy. Even though recent peer-reviewed literature includes numerous publications about the treatment of postoperative endophthalmitis, none of the papers offers a prospective, randomized study of modern, complete pars plana vitrectomy versus vitreous tap and intravitreal antibiotics only.

- A pretreatment vitreous tap for microbial analysis is always required and should be gained by a vitreous cutter.
- Inject 1 mg (0.1 cc) of vancomycin, 2.5 mg (0.1 cc) of ceftazidime, and 25 mg (0.1 cc) of prednisolone into the vitreous cavity with a 23-gauge needle.
- If there is no significant improvement in the clinical aspect of the eye a second intravitreal injection is administered on the third day.
- The causal bacteria seem to be the most important prognostic factor in endophthalmitis after cataract surgery.
- The production of bacterial exotoxins and increased microbial motility may lead to very early and severe functional damage even in the presence of only mild inflammation with a relatively small amount of bacteria. In such cases, any therapeutic intervention may be unsatisfactory and the visual outcome may commonly be poor.

6

6.1 Introduction

6.1.1 Basics

After cataract surgery, intraocular bacteria can be observed in as many as 29–43% of all patients without any pathologic response [7, 29]. A minority of these patients, however, develop an inflammatory reaction as a result of the colonization of bacteria or fungi, which gives the clinical impression of endophthalmitis. Exogenous endophthalmitis due to cataract surgery is rare and occurs in approximately 0.05% of all cases, with a growing incidence since the routine use of no-stitch cataract surgery began [20, 23, 34]. The risk of endophthalmitis is mainly dependent on the surgical technique used [24, 27, 32]; however, there is no evidence that the duration and complications of surgery as well as diabetes mellitus and immunosuppression will additionally increase the danger of developing endophthalmitis [30, 36]. As the extent of bacterial adhesion appears to depend on the specific lens material

used, the intraocular lens used seems to add to the specific risk of endophthalmitis [3, 16].

6.1.2 Pathophysiology

In most cases of intraoperative microbial contamination, protective mechanisms known as the anterior or posterior chamber-associated immune deviation (ACAID/POCAID) prevent eyes from disastrous inflammatory mechanisms [33]. Compromise of this "immune privilege" by intraoperative complications like capsular damage or vitreous loss can cause a 14-fold increased risk of endophthalmitis [19].

6.1.2.1 Phases of Infection

In infectious endophthalmitis, specific clinical phases can be distinguished [15], as illustrated in Fig. 6.1. These are dependent on the route of infection as well as on the type and virulence of the

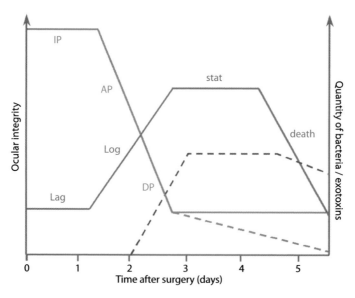

Fig. 6.1   Phases of bacterial growth and concurrent endophthalmitis development. The curves show an example of time-dependent intraocular bacterial growth and concurrent endophthalmitis development after cataract surgery. *Red line* ocular integrity/retinal function (*dotted* in the case of exotoxins); *green line* bacterial growth; *blue line* exotoxin release (if appropriate). In the late phase of acute endophthalmitis there is no functional recovery because of retinal damage despite bacterial cell death. The presence of exotoxins may add to severe ocular impairment. *IP* incubation phase, *AP* acceleration phase, *DP* destructive phase, *Lag* bacterial lag phase without increase in cell number, *Log* phase of exponential bacterial growth, *stat* stationary bacterial phase, *death* exponential bacterial death phase

inoculated microbes and the patients' immune state. Under unfortunate clinical conditions those phases will develop faster and the destructive power of the inflammation will be stronger.

6.1.2.1.1 Incubation Phase

The first step of exogenous endophthalmitis after cataract surgery is clinically unapparent and develops in the earliest postoperative period. It lasts at least 16–18 h even in patients with highly virulent pathogens. The generation time of the microbes is the main determinant for the duration of this phase.

6.1.2.1.2 Acceleration Phase

Dependent on the inoculated number and virulence of the microbes, endophthalmitis becomes symptomatic by breakdown of the blood–aqueous barrier. Increasing inflammatory reactions cause fibrin exudation and leukocyte migration into the anterior chamber and vitreous. These signs are predominantly accompanied by individual symptoms like visual loss and pain. The higher the virulence of the pathogen the earlier and the more serious the inflammatory response.

6.1.2.1.3 Destructive Phase

Destruction of retinal tissue is the catastrophic injury eventually leading to the bad functional outcome of endophthalmitis. The cytotoxic properties of some microbes, as well as the inflammation itself, may lead to substantial disorganization and necrosis of the retina [14, 18, 26]. If this phase of endophthalmitis is reached, the chance of successful treatment will diminish rapidly.

6.1.3 Clinical Diagnosis

Most of the patients with acute endophthalmitis after cataract surgery become symptomatic between 1 day and 2 weeks after surgery. Reduced vision after initially good visual acuity is present in virtually all of these cases [10, 35]. Table 6.1 lists the most important clinical signs arranged by their incidence. Figure 6.2 gives a representative illustration of acute postoperative endophthalmitis.

Table 6.1 Clinical symptoms of acute endophthalmitis after cataract surgery [10, 35]

Indicator	Remarks
Visual loss (>90%)	Blurred vision down to no perception of light within several hours and up to 1 day
Uveitis anterior (>90%)	Cloudy anterior chamber: cells, Tyndall sign and fibrin coagulate
Hypopyon (75–86%)	Concave to horizontal and smooth in bacterial infection; sometimes convex and spiky in fungal endophthalmitis
Pain (74–85%)	Moderate to heavy ocular pain, sometimes nausea
Ocular redness (>80%)	Pericorneal injection, later diffuse redness
Conjunctival chemosis	
Eyelid chemosis	
Vitritis	Sometimes with vitreous abscess and retinal edema or signs of retinitis
Absent red reflex	In the case of severe anterior or total vitritis
Corneal edema	Sometimes with infiltrates or ring abscess

6

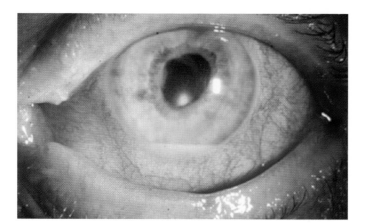

Fig. 6.2 Slit-lamp appearance of acute endophthalmitis

6.1.3.1 Role of Ultrasonography

In the case of opaque media, ophthalmic ultrasound may give valuable information about the clinical situation of the posterior segment in acute endophthalmitis. A recent ultrasonographic study of 137 eyes suggested that some echographic parameters might help to assess the functional outcome of infectious endophthalmitis [5]. There was a positive correlation between poor visual outcome and the presence of dense vitreous opacities and choroidal detachment. Furthermore, the authors found an association between the grade of vitreous opacity, choroidal detachment, and the causative group of bacteria. Longitudinal examination by ultrasound may also be useful to follow treatment effects and to decide whether additional therapy is needed in due course. The different echographic appearance of diverse microbes is illustrated in Figs. 6.3 and 6.4.

6.1.4 Microbial Spectrum

If a vitreous tap is taken, up to two-thirds of all cultures are expected to be positive and only in those cases is exact antibiotic therapy possible [12]. Hence, comprehensive information about the spectrum of microorganisms causing post-surgical endophthalmitis is necessary for the selection of appropriate antibiotic cocktails.

Gram-positive bacteria cause by far the most cases of acute endophthalmitis after cataract surgery. The number of Gram-negative cases is decreasing and current data suggest an incidence of considerably less than 10% [11]. A survey of studies investigating the microbiologic aspects of postoperative endophthalmitis reveals that co-agulase-negative staphylococci represent about half of all culture-positive acute endophthalmitis cases, followed by *Staphylococcus aureus* and β-hemolytic streptococci [1, 9, 11]. Figures 6.5–6.7 give an idea of the microbiologic view of endophthalmitis.

The frequent use of antibiotics in medicine has led to growing resistance of pathogens [17]. In endophthalmitis, bacteria have become increasingly resistant to ciprofloxacin and cefazolin, a tendency that may be caused by the growing preoperative use of fluoroquinolones [22].

Summary for the Clinician

- After cataract surgery the presence of bacteria in the anterior chamber is common.
- Postoperative endophthalmitis is rare and is maintained by surgical technique and patient-related risk factors.
- Visual loss in the early postoperative period is a warning symptom for endophthalmitis, even in the absence of pain.

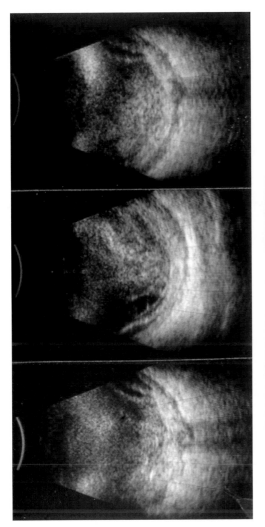

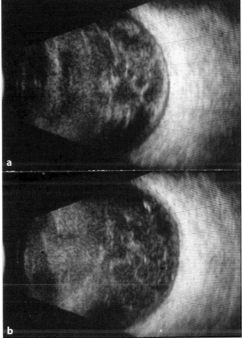

Fig. 6.3 Ocular echography of acute enterococcus endophthalmitis. Consecutive B-scans (10-MHz probe) of an eye with acute endophthalmitis due to enterococcus species within 2 days of phacoemulsification with IOL implantation are shown. *Top*: on echography several hours after the onset of symptoms severe intravitreal infiltrates and thickening of the choroidal layer are visible. Note that there is a "T-sign" due to increased fluid in the sub-Tenon space, which indicates the beginning of panophthalmitis. *Middle*: 1 day later the situation has worsened in spite of intravitreal antibiotics. There is major thickening of the choroid and the beginning of retinal detachment. *Bottom*: 5 days later diffuse panophthalmic infiltration is present despite a second intravitreal injection of specific antibiotics (courtesy of Dr. A.M. Verbeek, Nijmegen)

Fig. 6.4 Ocular echography of acute staphylococcus epidermidis endophthalmitis. Consecutive B-scans (10-MHz probe) of an eye with acute endophthalmitis because of *Staphylococcus epidermidis* are presented. **a** The initial echographic situation 3 days after phacoemulsification with IOL implantation shows moderate intravitreal membranes and infiltrates. **b** Four days later the situation has improved after a single intravitreal injection of ceftazidime and vancomycin. Note that the initial choroidal thickening has disappeared (courtesy of Dr. A.M. Verbeek, Nijmegen)

6

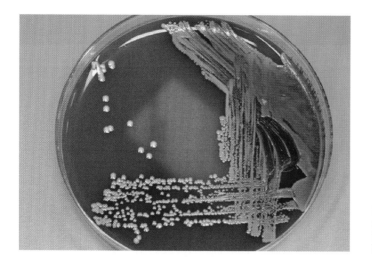

Fig. 6.5 Cultured coagulase-negative staphylococci (courtesy of Dr. T. Schülin-Casonato, Nijmegen)

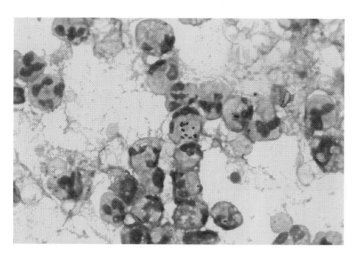

Fig. 6.6 Gram-positive staphylococci and granulocytes in a vitreous tap (courtesy of Dr. T. Schülin-Casonato, Nijmegen)

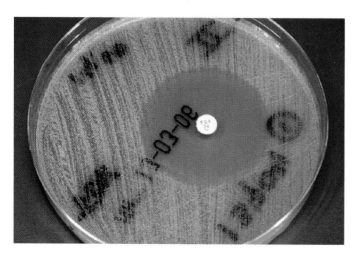

Fig. 6.7 Antibiotics sensitivity testing (courtesy of Dr. T. Schülin-Casonato, Nijmegen)

Summary for the Clinician

- The onset of symptoms mainly depends on the generation time of the causal microbe.
- About one-third of all vitreous taps in endophthalmitis remain culture-negative.
- The predominant microbes in endophthalmitis after cataract surgery are Gram-positive bacteria and among these, coagulase-negative staphylococci are the most common.
- The frequent preoperative use of antibiotics has led to growing bacterial resistance.

6.2 Therapeutical Approaches

6.2.1 Basics

When the diagnosis endophthalmitis has been made a medical emergency is present and the next diagnostic and therapeutic steps do not permit any delays. We strongly advise carrying out a vitreous tap and injecting antibiotics into the vitreous cavity within less than an hour of the clinical diagnosis. Only adequate treatment in the early hours of the disease may protect the eye from substantial inflammation of the posterior segment and might limit toxic bacterial damage.

To allow a specific treatment of the causal microbe it is important to obtain vitreous for Gram staining, microbial culture, and an antibiogram before the instillation of antibiotics. It is therefore essential to perform a vitreous tap immediately, independent of the availability of an operation theater or a specialized vitreoretinal surgeon. We advise against an anterior chamber puncture only, as pathogen identification from anterior chamber specimens is less successful. Corneal or conjunctival swabs are useless as well, as there is no convenient correlation between microbes found in those swabs and pathogens causative of the accompanying endophthalmitis [2, 31].

It is helpful to cooperate with a microbiologist to get reliable microscopy results of Gram-stained vitreous specimens within an hour. After 24 h the first findings of the microbiological cultures are available and antibiotic sensitivity testing is achievable within 6–48 h, depending on the method used [21]. Equal microbiologic results can be expected by samples obtained by a vitreous cutter or by needle aspiration [13].

6.2.2 Early Pars Plana Vitrectomy

Since the results of the Endophthalmitis Vitrectomy Study [10] have been published it has generally been believed that immediate pars plana vitrectomy (PPV) is not advantageous over simple intravitreal administration of antibiotics. However, some surgeons still prefer early PPV, possibly together with extraction of the intraocular lens implant, in the case of endophthalmitis after cataract surgery. Early PPV supports the ancient surgical principle of relieving an abscess immediately (“*Ubi pus, ibi evacua*”). On the other hand, vitreoretinal surgery in the severely inflamed endophthalmitis eye includes a number of significant risk factors.

First, there will be bad visibility caused by fibrin, cells, pus, synechia, corneal edema, and vitreous haze. Good visibility of the intraocular structures is crucial for safe PPV with a favorable surgical outcome. If PPV is performed early in endophthalmitis subtotal vitrectomy has to be achieved, which cannot be done safely with poor retinal visibility.

Second, the retina in cases of endophthalmitis is very fragile and possibly necrotic. Even though in the Endophthalmitis Vitrectomy Study retinal detachment in the vitrectomy group was as frequent as in the no vitrectomy group [8], in study patients no posterior vitreous separation and only a limited vitrectomy of "at least 50% of the vitreous" were carried out. In contrast, a PPV fulfilling the intention of total abscess removal with vitreous separation and shaving will probably lead to retinal tear formation and subsequent retinal detachment.

Third, in heavy inflammation like endophthalmitis the choroid is thickened and the ocular blood flow is increased. Together with poor visibility the latter enlarges the risk of choroidal detachment, sub-choroidal infusion and severe hemorrhages during surgery.

6

6.2.3 Nonvitrectomizing Endophthalmitis Treatment

As discussed before, early complete PPV includes several risks that may lead to worse surgical results compared with nonvitrectomized eyes. In patients with worst functional outcome the presence of motile toxin-producing microbes is likely [4, 14]. These toxins may seriously damage the retina within a few hours of the onset of symptoms. Removal of the microbes by PPV in such cases will not improve the retinal situation, but increase the risk of additional surgical damage. On the other hand, microorganisms that do not produce toxins will be much less harmful to the retina and the functional outcome is likely to be better. In such cases antibiotic blockage of the microbial reproduction will sufficiently limit the intraocular inflammation without the need for an additional early PPV.

Summary for the Clinician

■ Endophthalmitis is a medical emergency and treatment should be initiated within 1 h.
■ A pretreatment vitreous tap for microbial analysis is always required and should be obtained by a vitreous cutter.
■ Information about Gram-staining is available within 1 h whereas microbial culture needs at least 24 h.
■ Dependent on the microbiologic technique, an antibiogram can be obtained within 6–48 h.
■ Early pars plana vitrectomy in endophthalmitis has several limitations and should be avoided.

6.3 Emergency Management of Endophthalmitis After Cataract Surgery

6.3.1 Surgical Technique

Since prompt treatment of endophthalmitis is mandatory the procedure should be performed in an outpatient setting. Instill two drops of 1% tetracaine followed by a retrobulbar or sub-Tenon injection with 3–5 cc of 2% mepivacaine, preferably with 150 IE of hyaluronidase added to the anesthetic solution for better diffusion in the retrobulbar space. Since an eye with endophthalmitis is inflamed and often painful one should wait at least 5 min to let the anesthetic work. Disinfect the eyelid, lashes, and periocular skin with 10% povidone iodine swabs, starting with the eyelid followed by the lashes and skin. Make certain that the eyelid margins and lashes are swabbed, and proceed in a systematic fashion, from the medial to the temporal aspect. Place a sterile ophthalmic drape over the eye to isolate the operation field before placing a lid speculum. Instill two drops of 5% povidone iodine ophthalmic solution in the eye and wait for 2 min. Wearing gloves, create a stab incision with a 0.6 mm (23-gauge) MVR blade 4 mm posterior to the limbus at the temporal superior part of the eye, stabilizing the eye with Barraquer-Troutman forceps. After that, introduce the disposable vitrectome into the eye and while cutting let an assistant gently aspirate 0.1–0.3 cc of fluid from the vitreous cavity. Remove the vitrectome gently from the eye and aspirate all fluid remnants from the cutter. Then disconnect the syringe containing the biopsy material from the tubing and close it with a sterile cap and send the biopsy material immediately to the microbiology lab for Gram staining and culture. Inject 1 mg (0.1 cc) of vancomycin, 2.5 mg (0.1 cc) of ceftazidime and 25 mg (0.1 cc) of prednisolone with a 23-gauge needle into the vitreous cavity. Digitally, check the intraocular pressure and perform a paracentesis in the case of high pressure. After patching the eye the patient is hospitalized or alternatively sent home to be seen the next day in the case of an outpatient setting.

There is an ongoing debate about the additional effect of frequent topical treatment. At present, we prescribe topical gentamicin (22.5 mg/ml) eight times daily, topical cefazolin (33 mg/ml) eight times daily, and topical 0.1% dexamethasone four times daily. Patients are seen the next day and sometimes twice daily in the case of suspected progression of the endophthalmitis. If there is no significant improvement in the clinical aspect of the eye a second intravitreal injection is administered on the third day.

6.3.2 Equipment for the Emergency Management of Endophthalmitis

- Instruments (Fig. 6.8)
  - Eye speculum
  - Anatomical forceps
  - Irrigation cannula
  - Conjunctival scissors
  - Vitrectome hand piece and unit
  - Troutman-Barraquer forceps
- Disposables
  - Surgical drape
  - Sterile surgical gloves
  - 10% povidone iodine swabs
  - 5% povidone iodine solution
  - Three plastic cups
  - One syringe (6.0 cc)
  - Four syringes (1.0 cc)
  - Cotton tip applicators
  - Three 30-gauge needles
  - Three sterile caps for syringes
  - 4×4-cm sterile cotton pads
  - 23-gauge microvitreoretinal blade
  - Eye pad and tape
- Medication
  - 1% Tetracaine
  - 2% Mepivacaine
  - 150 IE Hyaluronidase
  - 0.1 cc Ceftazidime (22.5 mg/ml)
  - 0.1 cc Vancomycin (10 mg/ml)
  - 0.1 cc Prednisolone (25 mg/ml)

6.3.3 Treatment Protocol

After the clinical diagnosis of acute endophthalmitis immediate treatment within 1 h is essential to give the eye any chance to recover. It is important to inform the microbiologist earlier to get pathogen analysis without delay. As previously described, a 0.1–0.3 ml biopsy of infected vitreous is gained and sent to the laboratory for immediate Gram staining, culture, and antibiotic sensitivity testing. Figure 6.9 shows a treatment map for acute postoperative endophthalmitis as practiced at our department.

6.3.4 Treatment Outcome in Endophthalmitis Without Immediate Vitrectomy

6.3.4.1 Introduction

The treatment of acute postoperative endophthalmitis continues to be controversially discussed within the ophthalmologic literature. The Endophthalmitis Vitrectomy Study was a large, prospective, randomized study, which aimed to evaluate whether immediate, pars plana vitrectomy or a vitreous tap only plus intravitreal antibiotics with or without systemic antibiotics was more favorable in the management of acute postoperative endophthalmitis [10]. The authors of this study postulated that immediate vitrectomy and systemic antibiotics were not advantageous for eyes with visual acuity better than light perception. Since then, vitreoretinal specialists

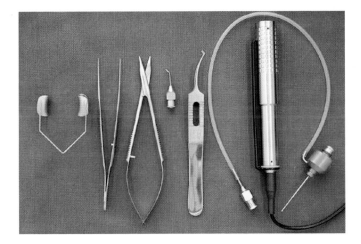

Fig. 6.8 Surgical instruments for emergency treatment of endophthalmitis

Fig. 6.9 Treatment strategy for acute endophthalmitis after cataract surgery

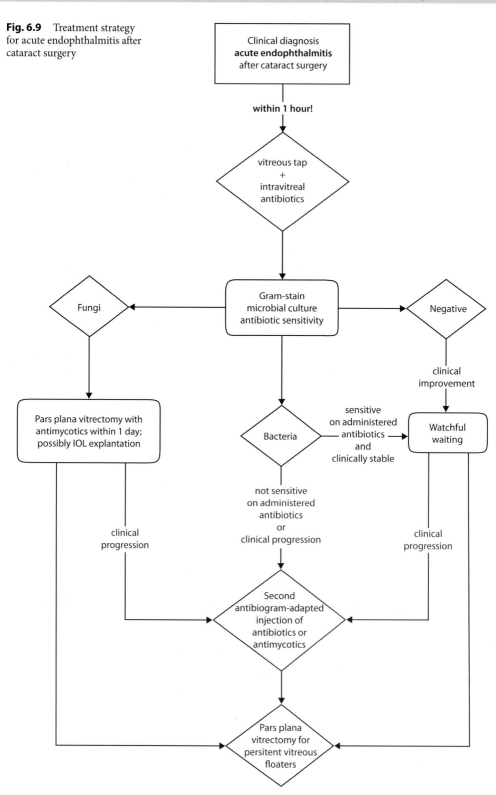

all over the world have been divided into two camps: those who avoided early vitrectomy and those who claimed the obligation of immediate complete pars plana vitrectomy. Even though recent peer-reviewed literature includes numerous publications on the treatment of postoperative endophthalmitis, none of the papers offers a prospective, randomized study of modern, complete pars plana vitrectomy versus vitreous tap and intravitreal antibiotics only.

Most patients with acute postoperative endophthalmitis will present in the phase of exponential bacterial growth ($n \times 2^t$) when bacteria will duplicate per time unit. That means, the earlier antibiotics are administered the less bacteria will be present in the eye and the more effective the antibiotic treatment will be. Intravitreal injection of potent antibiotics is the most effective way of reaching the greatest concentration of therapeutics in the eye. In addition, the simple surgical procedure of a pars plana injection after a vitreous tap can be performed as an office procedure, which guarantees rapid performance without time loss.

6.3.4.2 Results in Our Department

We analyzed 83 eyes of 83 patients treated in our department for acute infectious endophthalmitis following phacoemulsification between 1 January 1998 and 31 December 2004. All eyes had initial diagnostic vitrectomy and all were administered intravitreal antibiotics (vancomycin and ceftazidime) immediately, as described earlier. In 29 eyes (35%) intravitreal prednisolone was injected according to the physician's preference. Immediate three-port pars plana vitrectomy was not performed in any of the patients. If necessary, a second and third intravitreal injection of antibiotics was given, depending on the clinical course and bacterial sensitivity testing. All patients with positive microbiological testing had bacterial infections, and none had a fungal infection.

Pathogens could be cultured from the vitreous taps of 56 out 83 patients (67.5%), 52% of which were coagulase-negative staphylococci, 21.5% were streptococci, and 14% *Staphylococcus aureus*. Other pathogens found were *Pseudomonas aeroginosa*, *Enterococcus faecalis*, *Achromobacter xylosoxidans*, and *Haemophilus influenzae*. Streptococci (45.5%) were the most frequently found bacteria in eyes with bad visual outcome, followed by *Staphylococcus aureus* (27.3%).

There was a trend toward better visual recovery if the bacterial culture was negative; however, the difference was not statistically significant. Diabetes mellitus and the intravitreal administration of prednisolone did not appear to have a significant impact on the final visual outcome. The mean course of visual acuity in our patients is shown in Fig. 6.10. In our series, 59% of all patients gained a useful final visual acuity of 20/40 or more and 18% of all eyes ended up with 20/200 or less. In 21.7% of the eyes pars plana vitrectomy was performed in due course to treat vitreous floaters. Detailed clinical data on our patients are listed in Table 6.2.

Table 6.2 Data of patients with infectious endophthalmitis after cataract surgery treated in our department. *VA* visual acuity, *NLP* no light perception

Clinical data	Positive microbial culture	Negative microbial culture
Age (years)	73±10	69±15
Gender (male:female)	25:31	8:19
Diabetes mellitus	10.7%	7.4%
Initial VA all	20/400 (NLP–20/20)	20/400 (NLP–20/63)
Final VA all	20/40 (NLP–20/20)	20/40 (NLP–20/20)
Final VA diabetic patients	20/40 (20/800–20/20)	20/50 (20/100–20/32)
Final VA ≤20/200	19.6%	14.8%
Final VA ≥20/40	57.1%	66.7%
Interval of symptoms	2 (0–32) days	3 (0–13) days

6

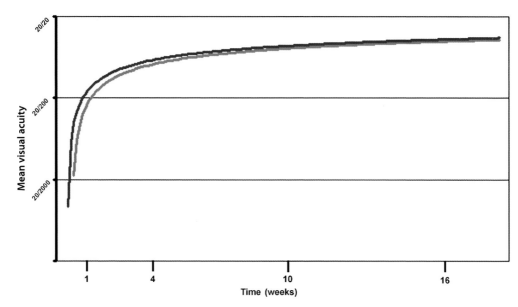

Fig. 6.10 The course of mean visual acuity after the treatment of infectious endophthalmitis by intravitreal antibiotics without complete pars plana vitrectomy. The exponential mean visual recovery over time in patients with infectious postoperative endophthalmitis treated at our department. The *red line* indicates patients with positive culture on a vitreous tap; the *blue line* represents patients with a negative vitreous tap

6.3.4.3 Discussion

The results of our study, as well as data from several other studies, suggest comparable outcomes of patients with acute postoperative endophthalmitis treated with a vitreous tap and intravitreal administration of antibiotics only [10, 25, 36]. There is no strong evidence of a general benefit of an early full pars plana vitrectomy in acute endophthalmitis. Data on the immediate intravitreal injection of steroids are discordant; however, there is a lack of prospective, randomized, placebo-controlled trials covering this issue [6, 12, 28]. It has been shown that infections with cytotoxic bacterial species lead to more severe retinal damage [14]. The production of bacterial exotoxins and increased microbial motility may lead to very early and severe functional damage, even in the presence of only mild inflammation with a relatively small amount of bacteria. In such cases, any therapeutical intervention may be unsatisfactory and the visual outcome may commonly be poor [4]. Providentially, noncytotoxic bacteria cause the bulk of acute endophthalmitis after cataract surgery, and intravitreal antibiotics alone can effectively be used in such cases. So far

there is no rationale for performing immediate three-port pars plana vitrectomy on eyes with acute bacterial postoperative endophthalmitis, as it may not improve the final visual outcome and this surgery is risky on an acutely inflamed eye.

Summary for the Clinician

- There is still no strong evidence whether immediate pars plana vitrectomy may be beneficial in acute postoperative endophthalmitis.
- Most patients gain final visual acuity of at least 20/40 after treatment with intravitreal antibiotics with no vitrectomy.
- In general, a significant number of patients will still have poor final visual acuity after postoperative endophthalmitis (<20/200).
- The causal bacteria seem to be the most important prognostic factor in endophthalmitis after cataract surgery.
- Thus far, the value of an additional intravitreal injection of steroids is unclear.

6.4 Conclusion

Infectious endophthalmitis is probably the most devastating complication of modern cataract surgery. In this chapter, we discuss the management of acute endophthalmitis after cataract surgery and give advice in the light of the existing literature data and our own results.

Most cases of endophthalmitis become apparent in the early postoperative period and immediate treatment is mandatory to circumvent avoidable ocular damage. Acute visual loss and pain together with uveitis and hypopyon are the most prominent clinical signs in eyes with acute postoperative endophthalmitis. Ophthalmic ultrasound can give useful additional prognostic information and should be performed if available.

Within the last decade the rising amount of infectious endophthalmitis after cataract surgery suggests a higher risk for patients with sutureless clear corneal incisions, the predominant incision technique in current cataract surgery. Most cases of acute endophthalmitis are caused by Gram-positive, coagulase-negative staphylococci, followed by *Staphylococcus aureus*, and β-hemolytic streptococci. Fungi are still important pathogens, and may be responsible for up to 8% of all postoperative endophthalmitides.

Acute endophthalmitis after cataract surgery is a medical emergency and urgent therapeutical steps have to be taken as soon as the clinical diagnosis has been made. A vitreous tap has to be performed immediately with a vitreous cutter via pars plana to gain material for microbiological cultures and sensitivity testing. Directly after that, an antibiotic cocktail of vancomycin and ceftazidime or amikacin must be injected intravitreally through the same incision. As soon as the microbiological results are available, a second, pathogen-adapted, intravitreal injection of antibiotics may be administered.

To date, there has been no strong evidence that early, full three-port pars plana vitrectomy in acute postoperative endophthalmitis may improve the final functional outcome. In contrast, complete vitrectomy with creation of a posterior vitreous detachment and cutting of the vitreous base may carry several serious risks in acute endophthalmitis. Our results, together with the literature data, suggest that early complete vitrec-

tomy is not superior to a vitreous tap with antibiotics only and consequently should be avoided. The rapid intravitreal injection of broad-spectrum antibiotics following a vitreous tap is the most critical therapeutical step to be taken in this disastrous postoperative complication.

Acknowledgements

The authors are grateful to Dr. A.M. Verbeek for expert echographic advice and for the use of Figs. 6.3 and 6.4, to N. Crama for data analysis of endophthalmitis patients, and to Dr. T. Schülin-Casonato for the use of Figs. 6.5–6.7.

References

1. Aaberg TM Jr, Flynn HW Jr, Schiffman J, et al. (1998) Nosocomial acute-onset postoperative endophthalmitis survey. A 10-year review of incidence and outcomes. Ophthalmology 105:1004–1010

2. Barza M, Pavan PR, Doft BH, et al. (1997) Evaluation of microbiological diagnostic techniques in postoperative endophthalmitis in the Endophthalmitis Vitrectomy Study. Arch Ophthalmol 115:1142–1150

3. Burillon C, Kodjikian L, Pellon G, et al. (2002) In-vitro study of bacterial adherence to different types of intraocular lenses. Drug Dev Ind Pharm 28:95–99

4. Callegan MC, Kane ST, Cochran DC, et al. (2005) Bacillus endophthalmitis: roles of bacterial toxins and motility during infection. Invest Ophthalmol Vis Sci 46:3233–3238

5. Dacey MP, Valencia M, Lee MB, et al. (1994) Echographic findings in infectious endophthalmitis. Arch Ophthalmol 112:1325–1333

6. Das T, Jalali S, Gothwal VK, et al. (1999) Intravitreal dexamethasone in exogenous bacterial endophthalmitis: results of a prospective randomised study. Br J Ophthalmol 83:1050–1055

7. Dickey JB, Thompson KD, Jay WM. (1991) Anterior chamber aspirate cultures after uncomplicated cataract surgery. Am J Ophthalmol 112:278–282

8. Doft BM, Kelsey SF, Wisniewski SR. (2000) Retinal detachment in the endophthalmitis vitrectomy study. Arch Ophthalmol 118:1661–1665

6

9. Driebe WT Jr, Mandelbaum S, Forster RK, et al. (1986) Pseudophakic endophthalmitis. Diagnosis and management. Ophthalmology 93:442–448

10. Endophthalmitis Vitrectomy Study Group. (1995) Results of the Endophthalmitis Vitrectomy Study. A randomized trial of immediate vitrectomy and of intravenous antibiotics for the treatment of postoperative bacterial endophthalmitis. Arch Ophthalmol 113:1479–1496

11. Endophthalmitis Vitrectomy Study Group. (1996) Microbiologic factors and visual outcome in the Endophthalmitis Vitrectomy Study. Am J Ophthalmol 122:830–846

12. Gan IM, Ugahary LC, van Dissel JT, et al. (2005) Intravitreal dexamethasone as adjuvant in the treatment of postoperative endophthalmitis: a prospective randomized trial. Graefes Arch Clin Exp Ophthalmol 243:1200–1205

13. Han DP, Wisniewski SR, Kelsey SF, et al. (1999) Microbiologic yields and complication rates of vitreous needle aspiration versus mechanized vitreous biopsy in the Endophthalmitis Vitrectomy Study. Retina 19:98–102

14. Jett BD, Jensen HG, Atkuri RV, et al. (1995) Evaluation of therapeutic measures for treating endophthalmitis caused by isogenic toxin-producing and toxin-nonproducing Enterococcus faecalis strains. Invest Ophthalmol Vis Sci 36:9–15

15. Kain HL. (1997) [Basic principles in treatment of endophthalmitis] (in German). Klin Monatsbl Augenheilkd 210:274–288

16. Kodjikian L, Burillon C, Chanloy C, et al. (2002) In vivo study of bacterial adhesion to five types of intraocular lenses. Invest Ophthalmol Vis Sci 43:3717–3721

17. Livermore DM. (2005) Minimising antibiotic resistance. Lancet Infect Dis 5:450–459

18. Maxwell DP Jr, Brent BD, Diamond JG, et al. (1991) Effect of intravitreal dexamethasone on ocular histopathology in a rabbit model of endophthalmitis. Ophthalmology 98:1370–1375

19. Menikoff JA, Speaker MG, Marmor M, et al. (1991) A case-control study of risk factors for postoperative endophthalmitis. Ophthalmology 98:1761–1768

20. Miller JJ, Scott IU, Flynn HW Jr, et al. (2005) Acute-onset endophthalmitis after cataract surgery (2000–2004): incidence, clinical settings, and visual acuity outcomes after treatment. Am J Ophthalmol 139(6):983–987

21. Mino de Kaspar H, Neubauer AS, Molnar A, et al. (2002) Rapid direct antibiotic susceptibility testing in endophthalmitis. Ophthalmology 109:687–693

22. Mino de Kaspar H, Shriver EM, Nguyen EV, et al. (2003) Risk factors for antibiotic-resistant conjunctival bacterial flora in patients undergoing intraocular surgery. Graefes Arch Clin Exp Ophthalmol 241:730–733

23. Montan PG, Koranyi G, Setterquist HE, et al. (1998) Endophthalmitis after cataract surgery: risk factors relating to technique and events of the operation and patient history: a retrospective case-control study. Ophthalmology 105:2171–2177

24. Nagaki Y, Hayasaka S, Kadoi C, et al. (2003) Bacterial endophthalmitis after small-incision cataract surgery. Effect of incision placement and intraocular lens type. J Cataract Refract Surg 29:20–26

25. Okhravi N, Towler HM, Hykin P, et al. (1997) Assessment of a standard treatment protocol on visual outcome following presumed bacterial endophthalmitis. Br J Ophthalmol 81:719–725

26. Peyman GA, Herbst R. (1974) Bacterial endophthalmitis. Treatment with intraocular injection of gentamicin and dexamethasone. Arch Ophthalmol 91:416–418

27. Schmitz S, Dick HB, Krummenauer F, et al. (1999) Endophthalmitis in cataract surgery: results of a German survey. Ophthalmology 106:1869–1877

28. Shah GK, Stein JD, Sharma S, et al. (2000) Visual outcomes following the use of intravitreal steroids in the treatment of postoperative endophthalmitis. Ophthalmology 107:486–489

29. Sherwood DR, Rich WJ, Jacob JS, et al. (1989) Bacterial contamination of intraocular and extraocular fluids during extracapsular cataract extraction. Eye 3:308–312

30. Somani S, Grinbaum A, Slomovic AR. (1997) Postoperative endophthalmitis: incidence, predisposing surgery, clinical course and outcome. Can J Ophthalmol 32:303–310

31. Speaker MG, Milch FA, Shah MK, et al. (1991) Role of external bacterial flora in the pathogenesis of acute postoperative endophthalmitis. Ophthalmology 98:639–649

32. Stonecipher KG, Parmley VC, Jensen H, et al. (1991) Infectious endophthalmitis following sutureless cataract surgery. Arch Ophthalmol 109:1562–1563

33. Streilein JW. (1996) Ocular immune privilege and the Faustian dilemma. The Proctor lecture. Invest Ophthalmol Vis Sci 37:1940–1950

34. Taban M, Behrens A, Newcomb RL, et al. (2005) Acute endophthalmitis following cataract surgery: a systematic review of the literature. Arch Ophthalmol 123:613–620

35. Wisniewski SR, Capone A, Kelsey SF, et al. (2000) Characteristics after cataract extraction or secondary lens implantation among patients screened for the Endophthalmitis Vitrectomy Study. Ophthalmology 107:1274–1282

36. Wu PC, Kuo HK, Li M, et al. (2005) Nosocomial postoperative endophthalmitis: a 14-year review. Graefes Arch Clin Exp Ophthalmol 14:1–10

Chapter 7

New Instruments in Vitrectomy

7

Masahito Ohji, Yasuo Tano

Core Messages

■ Development of new instruments has improved the outcomes of vitreous surgery.

■ Machemer developed the 17-gauge one-port vitrectomy system in 1971.

■ O'Malley and Heinz developed the three port vitrectomy system in 1972.

■ Recently, the 25-gauge vitrectomy system has been developed by Fujii, de Juan and colleagues.

■ One advantage of small-gauge vitrectomy is the small wound size, which is expected to be less invasive.

■ By using the trocar system, the surgeon can keep the scleral wound and the conjunctiva relatively intact.

■ The residual vitreous around the ora serata plugs the scleral wound.

■ The sutureless wound increases patient comfort postoperatively, which is another big advantage of small-gauge surgery.

■ The efficiency of removal of the vitreous is less in the 25-gauge vitrectomy system compared with the regular 20-gauge system.

■ Xenon light source that can provide bright illumination through a narrow light pipe is required.

7.1 Introduction

Since Machemer introduced the pars plana vitrectomy in 1971 [26], various kinds of instruments have been developed for vitreous surgery and have improved the outcome. For example, Machemer developed the 17-gauge one-port vitrectomy system using a full-function vitreous cutter including infusion cannula. He performed vitrectomy under slit-lamp illumination. O'Malley and Heinz then developed the three-port vitrectomy system in 1972, which is essentially the same system we are currently using [31]. There are other instruments that have made a breakthrough, including the laser system, fluid–air exchange, long-acting gas, silicone oil, and heavy liquid [1, 7, 8, 13, 32]. Recently, the 25-gauge vitrectomy system was developed by Fujii, de Juan and colleagues [14], followed by the similar innovation of the 23-gauge system developed by Eckardt [10]. Another breakthrough is the bright illumination system with a xenon light source that can provide bright illumination through a narrow light pipe as in the 25-gauge system. It allows the surgeon to carry out vitrectomy with the 25-gauge system and to use truly bi-manual techniques in the regular 20-gauge system.

7.2 Sutureless Transconjunctival Vitrectomy

7.2.1 25-Gauge Vitrectomy System

The specific features of Fujii et al.'s system include instruments with the 25-gauge, transconjunctival trocar system and sutureless wounds. The new instruments used in the new 25-gauge vitrectomy system are much smaller than the regular 20-gauge instruments. The advantage of small-gauge vitrectomy is the small wound size, which is expected to be less invasive. The second specific feature is the transconjunctival trocar system. The trocar system itself has been used in the regular 20-gauge system by some surgeons as well; however, it was not essential. Insertion of trocars through the conjunctiva and the sclera is the second specific feature and the key to the 25-gauge vitrectomy system. By using trocars, the surgeon can keep the wound relatively intact and intact scleral and conjunctival wounds are the key to the sutureless wound, which is the third feature. The residual vitreous around the ora serata also plays an important role by plugging the scleral wound. The sutureless wound increases patient comfort postoperatively, which is one of the biggest advantages of the surgery.

7.2.2 Instruments

Various kinds of instruments for 25-gauge vitrectomy have been developed. The trocars, the light pipes and the vitreous cutter are the essential instruments in every operation. Other instruments have also become available [14].

7.2.2.1 Trocars

The trocars (Fig. 7.1) are essential for the 25-gauge sutureless trans-conjunctival vitrectomy system, while some surgeons have even used trocars in the 20-gauge system. It is quite difficult to insert and pull out instruments through both the conjunctiva and the sclera without the trocar system. It also plays a key role in minimizing damage to the wound. This is essential to prevent leakage of fluid.

7.2.2.2 Vitreous Cutter

There are two different kinds of vitreous cutter (Fig. 7.2), the pneumatic cutter driven by air-pressure and the motor-driven cutter. Each has its advantages and disadvantages. The pneumatic cutter driven by air-pressure is light and has minimal vibration, while the motor-driven one has more precise control of the blade mo-

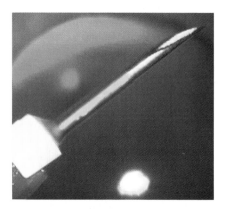

Fig. 7.1   25-gauge system trocars

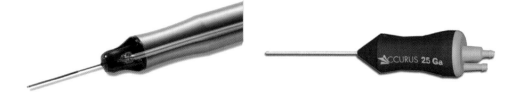

a   b

Fig. 7.2   25-gauge system vitreous cutter driven by **a** a motor and **b** by air-pressure

tions. Recently developed cutters have a maximum cutting speed limit of as fast as 2,500 rpm as in the 20-gauge system. Because of the narrow aperture of the vitreous cutter, the aspiration rate is smaller than that of the 20-gauge cutter. Therefore, the aspiration vacuum is usually set to 500–600 mmHg instead of 200 mmHg to achieve enough aspiration flow [15].

7.2.2.3 Light Pipe

The light pipe in the 25-gauge vitrectomy system is narrower than that in the 20-gauge vitrectomy system, and the 25-gauge light pipe connected to the regular illumination source offers dim illumination and does not allow visualization of the details of the fundus lesions. A combination of brighter light source and a good reflector is very important to achieve a better illumination system. The xenon light source can provide a much brighter light than a regular halogen light source and a spherical reflector can introduce uniform illumination without a dark spot in the center of the output pattern, as in the illumination system with a parabolic reflector (Fig. 7.3) The xenon light system provides very bright illumination through a narrow 25-gauge light pipe, which facilitates visualization of the details of the fundus lesions. This advance makes the 25-gauge vitrectomy system easier, more efficient, and safer, and increases the indications for 25-gauge vitrectomy.

7.2.2.4 Other 25-Gauge Instruments

Many other instruments, including the diathermy probe, laser probes, extendable curved pick, aspirating pick, various kinds of forceps, vertical scissors, curved scissors, and silicone-tipped blushed back-flush needles, have become available (Figs. 7.4, 7.5).

7.2.2.5 Other Instruments

The pressure plate developed by Eckardt is a special instrument for displacing the conjunctiva and inserting the trocars into the appropriate position (Fig. 7.6) [10]. It was developed for the 23-gauge system; however, it is useful in the 25-gauge system as well. The forceps with scale marks have two scale marks on the top surface and a serrated undersurface of the tip and can be used in a similar fashion (Fig. 7.7) [30]. The distance between the two scale marks is 4 mm and can be used for accurate measurement and the serrated under surface is useful for pulling the conjunctiva.

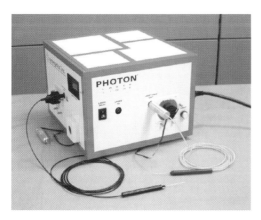
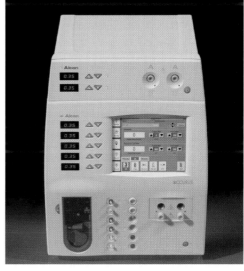

Fig. 7.3 Xenon light source. Both can provide enough illumination for detailed observation in the 25-gauge system

7

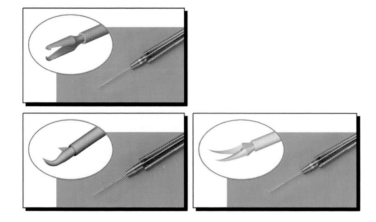

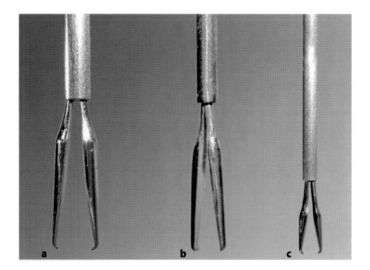

Fig. 7.4 The forceps, the vertical scissors, and the curved scissors

Fig. 7.5 Comparison of **a** 20-gauge, **b** 23-gauge, and **c** 25-gauge forceps

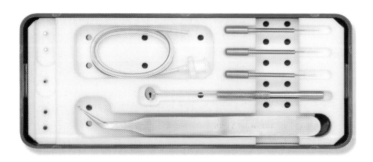

Fig. 7.6 Pressure plate

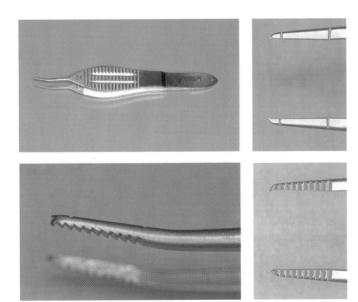

Fig. 7.7 Forceps with scale marks

7.2.3 Surgical Procedures of the 25-Gauge System

7.2.3.1 Insert Three Trocars

The conjunctiva should be pulled when the trocars are inserted into the sclera. The straight conduits of the scleral wound and the conjunctival wound may increase the risk of postoperative infection. Therefore, it is extremely important to displace the conjunctiva when trocars are inserted into the sclera through the conjunctiva to prevent straight conduits [15, 23]. It is also important to insert the trocars into the appropriate position, usually 3.5–4 mm from the limbus, in 25-gauge vitrectomy as well as in 20-gauge vitrectomy. The conjunctiva can be pulled and the trocars can be inserted in the appropriate position without a caliper using the pressure plate or the forceps with scale marks [10, 30]. The trocars are usually inserted perpendicularly to the sclera while some surgeons insert the trocars obliquely to improve sealing of the wounds.

7.2.3.2 Vitrectomy

The vitreous can be removed by the 25-gauge vitrectomy cutter. The removal of the vitreous is less efficient in the 25-gauge vitrectomy system compared with that with the regular 20-gauge system. To improve the efficiency, the suction should be set at 500–600 mmHg, which is much higher than in the regular 20-gauge system [15].

7.2.3.3 Closure of the Wound

The trocars are removed at the end of the surgery. The peripheral vitreous presumably plugs the scleral wound and no fluid leakage usually occurs without sutures in most cases. A gentle massage of the wound with a cotton swab or injection of a small amount of air may be useful to prevent fluid leakage from the wound, while a suture may be required to stop leakage in some cases [23].

7.2.4 Advantage and Disadvantage of 25-Gauge System

"Sutureless" wounds are one of the most important features of the 25-gauge system. Patients feel more comfortable following 25-gauge sutureless vitrectomy because there are no sutures on the ocular surface. Sutureless wounds obviously shorten surgical time and decrease the cost [14]. Another technique specific to the 25-gauge system is removing proliferative membranes with a vitreous cutter. The aperture of the vitrectomy cutter is closer to the tip of the vitreous cutter in the 25-gauge system compared with the 20-gauge system, allowing the surgeon to remove most of the membrane with a 25-gauge vitreous cutter without performing delamination using scissors.

The 25-gauge sutureless system also has several disadvantages, although dim illumination had already been resolved with the bright xenon illumination. The time needed for complete vitrectomy in the 25-gauge system may be longer than in the 20-gauge system because of the smaller aperture of the vitreous cutter, while total surgical time for selected cases could be shorter in the 25-gauge system [14]. The aspiration rate is lower in the 25-gauge system even if the aspiration pressure is set to 500–600 mmHg compared with that in the 20-gauge system [14]. The shafts of the instruments used during 25-gauge vitrectomy are much softer than those of the 20-gauge instruments [14]. When using 25-gauge instruments, it might be difficult to rotate the eyeball because the instruments are so soft. Small saccadic eye movements can be reduced using 20-gauge instruments, while it may be difficult to reduce saccadic eye movements sufficiently with 25-gauge instruments during fine maneuvers including removal of epiretinal membranes or internal limiting membranes in some cases. The 25-gauge instruments have become stiffer and likely will become more so in the future, and they will probably eventually be used just like 20-gauge instruments.

7.3 23-Gauge Vitrectomy System

Eckardt developed the 23-gauge vitrectomy system (Fig. 7.6) [10]. The 23-gauge system is similar to the 25-gauge system in many respects, while there are some differences. The 23-gauge trocars are made of steel and are re-usable, although disposable ones have become available recently. The trocars in the 23-gauge system are inserted obliquely following the use of the microvitreoretinal blade. An oblique pathway of the wound is essential to prevent fluid leakage because the scleral and conjunctival wound is obviously larger in the 23-gauge system than that

in 25-gauge system. The infusion and aspiration rates are higher in the 23-gauge system than in the 25-gauge system. The shaft of the 23-gauge instruments is much stiffer and can be used just like the 20-gauge instruments.

Summary for the Clinician

- The new instruments used in the new 25-gauge vitrectomy system are much smaller than the regular 20-gauge instruments
- Insertion of trocars through the conjunctiva and the sclera is the second specific feature and the key to the 25-gauge vitrectomy system.
- Because of the narrow aperture of the vitreous cutter, the aspiration rate is smaller than that of 20-gauge cutter. Therefore, the aspiration vacuum is usually set to 500–600 mmHg instead of 200 mmHg to achieve sufficient aspiration flow [15].
- The pressure plate was developed by Eckardt for 23-gauge system; however, it is useful in the 25-gauge system as well.
- It is extremely important to displace the conjunctiva when trocars are inserted into the sclera through the conjunctiva to prevent straight conduits.
- The peripheral vitreous presumably plug the scleral wound and no fluid leakage usually occurs without sutures in most cases.
- When using 25-gauge instruments, it might be difficult to rotate the eyeball because of the softness of the instruments. It may also be difficult to reduce saccadic eye movements sufficiently during fine maneuvers.

7.4 Xenon Endo-Illumination for Vitrectomy

Endo-illumination is one of the most important among the many kinds of instruments used during vitreous surgery and very bright endo-illumination without light hazard is extremely important. Recently, a bright illumination system using a xenon light source was developed.

The light pipe in the vitrectomy with the 25-gauge system is narrower than that in the regular 20-gauge vitrectomy system and the 25-gauge light pipe connected to the regular illumination source can offer dim illumination and does not allow surgeons to see the details of the fundus lesions. A brighter endo-illumination system would be essential to allow surgeons to see the details of the fundus lesions in the 25-gauge system. Very bright endo-illumination systems have been introduced by both Synergetics and Alcon (Fig. 7.3) Both illumination systems have a xenon light source and provide very bright illumination through the narrow 25-gauge light pipe that allows surgeons to visualize the details of the fundus lesions. It makes the 25-gauge vitrectomy system easier, more efficient, and safer, and increases the indications for 25-gauge vitrectomy. In addition to the light source, a reflector system is a major factor in providing brighter illumination. The xenon light source can shine a brighter light than the regular halogen light source and a spherical reflector plays an important role in introducing the bright light to the light fiber. It has a complex design with expensive optics; however, it can introduce uniform illumination without a dark spot in the center of the output pattern, as in the illumination system with a parabolic reflector.

The chandelier system has been available for long time; however, its usefulness was limited because of insufficient illumination. The 25-gauge chandelier illumination system is another instrument that became useful following the introduction of the bright xenon light source (Fig. 7.8). It allows surgeons to remove peripheral vitreous or to apply laser into the peripheral retina with scleral indentation when it is inserted into the trocar in the 25-gauge system. The illuminated infusion cannula is also useful when connected to the xenon light source, although the illuminated infusion cannula has been available with dim illumination (Fig. 7.9).

The new light source is also useful in the 20-gauge system. The chandelier illumination that is used as the fourth port allows surgeons to perform truly bi-manual techniques with the regular 20-gauge instruments. The bi-manual technique is useful and almost essential for treating complicated cases such as severe proliferative diabetic retinopathy or severe proliferative vitreoretinopathy; however, it required additional instruments including illuminated forceps and scissors. The illuminated instruments are extremely fragile and it is difficult to maintain them in a good condition. The 25-gauge chandelier illumination system allows the surgeon to use any of hundreds of regular 20-gauge instruments including forceps, scissors, diathermy, aspiration needle, and laser probes.

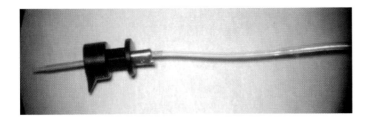

Fig. 7.8 25-gauge chandelier illumination

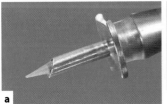
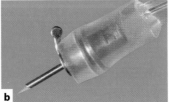

Fig. 7.9 **a** 20-gauge and **b** 25-gauge illuminated infusion cannula. The diameter of the light fiber is 500 um and 380 um respectively

7

7.4.1 Yellow-Filtered Xenon

Xenon light source can provide brighter light than the regular halogen light source, but the light provided by xenon contains more blue components. Subjects illuminated by the xenon light look whiter or paler compared with the halogen light. In addition to looking pale, we also have to pay attention to the light hazard caused by the blue components of the light. Light with a wavelength shorter than 550 nm is very hazardous for the retina; therefore, the blue components of wavelengths shorter than 550 nm have to be cut by a filter (Fig. 7.10). By cutting the blue components of the wavelength shorter than 550 nm, the safety of the retina is dramatically improved approximately 8-fold (Table 7.1).

Table 7.1 Hazard efficacy (lumens/hazard Watt). A higher number is safer

Light	Hazard efficacy (Lm/hazard Watt)
Xenon	1,913
Xenon with yellow filter	16,568
Halogen	1,920
Metal halide	1,343

7.4.2 Wide-Angle Viewing System

A wide-angle viewing system using a binocular indirect ophthalmomicroscope (BIOM) or contact lens has become popular because the surgeon can see a wider area of the fundus simultaneously (Fig. 7.11) [37]. By viewing a wider area of the fundus, the surgeon can recognize the fundus pathology better and can treat lesions more safely and efficiently. The focus of the new BIOM system can be adjusted by the surgeon using a foot-pedal, while the focus needs to be adjusted by a handle in the old BIOM model. The new contact lens for a wide angle viewing system has a smaller diameter (Fig. 7.12) [28]. The reduction of the diameter of the lens has made it possible to visualize the scleral port directly so that the insertion of surgical instruments through the scleral port can be accomplished without any problems.

An optical fiber-free intravitreal surgery system (OFFISS) is a new wide-angle viewing system combined with a surgical microscope (Fig. 7.13) [17]. The new system is similar to the BIOM system; however, there are some advantages. Surgeons can see the fundus with illumination incorporated into the microscope without using a light pipe. Therefore, it allows surgeons to perform a bimanual technique with regular instruments. Secondly, the surgeon can adjust the focus using the foot-pedal of the microscope, just

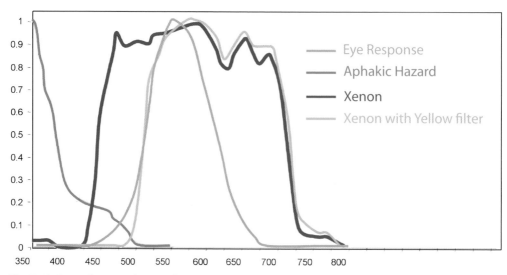

Fig. 7.10 Spectral output of xenon illumination and xenon illumination with yellow filter. By cutting the blue components, the safety of the xenon light is improved

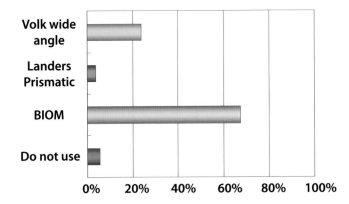

Fig. 7.11 Preferred wide-angle viewing system from the Practices and Trends (PAT) survey by the American Society of Retina Specialists. *BIOM* binocular indirect ophthalmo-microscope

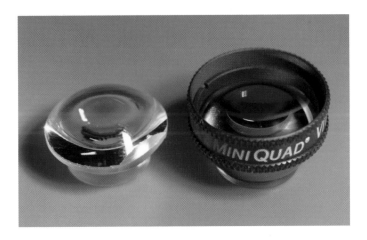

Fig. 7.12 ClariVit, a new wide-angle viewing contact lens with smaller diameter (*left*) than the regular wide-angle viewing contact lens (*right*)

like focusing under visualization using contact lens, and he or she has to adjust the focus using a foot-pedal or a focus ring that is different from the foot-pedal of the microscope in the BIOM.

An inverter is essential when it is used for the wide-angle viewing system including the BIOM or when the contact lens is used. The Inverter-tube is a new inverter that is incorporated into the Zeiss microscope (Fig. 7.14). The advantage of the new inverter is the shorter working distance between the eyes and the hands compared with previous inverters. Another advantage of the Invertertube is the better quality of inverted images. The Invertertube needs only one switchable prism to invert images, while a large number of prisms were needed to invert images in previous inverters. The simple mechanism produces better quality inverted images.

Summary for the Clinician

- The light pipe in the 25-gauge system is narrower than that in the regular 20-gauge vitrectomy system.
- Synergetics and Alcon manufacture xenon light sources that provide very bright illumination, even through the 25-gauge light pipe.
- The 25-gauge chandelier illumination system became useful following the introduction of the bright xenon light source.
- The chandelier illumination that is used as the fourth port allows surgeons to perform truly bi-manual techniques.
- It is also useful in the 20-gauge system.

7

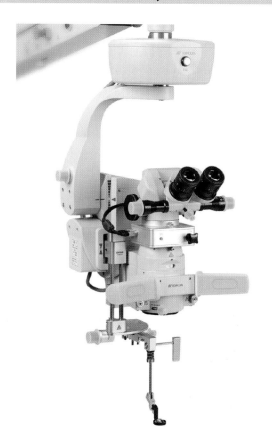

Fig. 7.13 Optical fiber-free intravitreal surgery system (OFFISS)

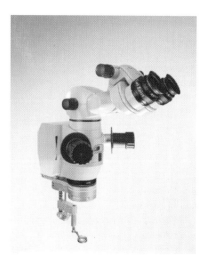

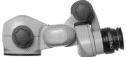

Fig. 7.14 The Invertertube

Summary for the Clinician

- By cutting the blue components of the wavelength shorter than 550 nm (yellow-filtered xenon), the safety of the retina is dramatically improved approximately 8-fold.
- The optical fiber-free intravitreal surgery system (OFFISS) is a new wide-angle viewing system attached to the surgical microscope.
- Surgeons can see the fundus without using a light pipe.
- It allows surgeons to use a bimanual technique with regular instruments

Table 7.2 Favorable reports of indocyanine green (ICG)-assisted inner limiting membrane (ILM) peeling in macular holes (MH). *VA* visual acuity

Reference	MH closure (%)	Improved VA (%)
[18]	92	84
[22]	88	59
[39]	97	62
[36]	97	71
[9]	98	96
[30]	95	82
Total	96	79

Table 7.3 Unfavorable reports of ICG-assisted ILM peeling in MH

Reference	MH closure (%)	Improved VA (%)
[11]	86	35
[16]	No data	55
[2]	100	25

7.4.3 Adjuncts

7.4.3.1 Staining of Internal Limiting Membrane with Indocyanine Green

Brooks reported internal limiting membrane (ILM) peeling for macular hole (MH) surgery in 1995 and achieved an improvement in anatomical and functional results [4]. ILM peeling has not been widely performed, however, because ILM peeling is technically difficult due to poor visibility of the ILM. Indocyanine green (ICG)-staining of ILM makes ILM peeling much easier and more complete [5, 18].

There are several reports with favorable results following ICG-assisted ILM peeling. Meta-analysis of these reports showed MH closure after initial surgery in 96% and improved visual acuity in 79% (Table 7.2) [18, 19–23]. On the other hand, there are also reports with unfavorable results (Table 7.3) [2, 11, 16]. Visual field defects could be one of the postoperative complications following ICG-assisted ILM peeling for MH or epiretinal membrane [16, 19]. Kanda et al. found that visual field defects were strongly related to the concentration of ICG [19]. When they stained ILM with 0.5% ICG for 3 min during MH surgery, visual field defects developed in all 12 eyes. They changed their technique to the injection of 0.5% ICG followed by immediate aspiration of ICG. With this technique, visual field defects developed in 1 out of 4 eyes. Then they diluted ICG more and used 0.25% ICG with immediate aspiration and did not find any visual field defects. Therefore, ICG is potentially toxic; however, this can be prevented or minimized by the appropriate use of ICG.

7.4.3.2 Other Dyes Staining the ILM

There are some alternatives to ICG. Trypan blue (0.3%) can be used to stain ILM; however, staining is weaker than ICG, while it stains the proliferative membrane well [12, 24]. Triamcinolone acetonide (TA) is one of the corticosteroids and is currently used to visualize the vitreous during vitrectomy [29, 31]. It is useful to see the vitreous

7

and it is almost impossible to detect the thin layer of vitreous cortex without TA, especially in highly myopic eyes. It has also been used to visualize the internal limiting membrane [20]. TA does not stain the ILM, but sits on the ILM and allows the surgeon to see it [33, 34].

7.4.3.2.1 Microplasmin

Plasmin is an enzyme that may be useful for pharmacological vitrectomy. It has been used for vitrectomy in traumatic pediatric macular holes and diabetic retinopathy [3, 27, 38]. It has also been shown that plasmin helps separate the vitreous hyaloid from the ILM surface in patients with diabetic retinopathy [3]. Microplasmin, which is a fragment of plasmin, may also be useful for pharmacological vitrectomy [35].

7.4.3.2.2 Perfluorocarbon Liquid and Heavy Silicone Oil

Perfluorocarbon liquid (PFCL) is a liquid that is heavier than water and has been used to reattach the retina during surgery. It is crucial to treat retinal detachment due to a giant tear or complicated vitreoretinopathy and macular translocation [6, 25]. PFCL cannot be used as a tamponade agent in the long term and has to be removed at the end of surgery because tamponading for long periods causes severe damage to the retina.

Perfluorohexyloctane is a semifluorinated alkane and its gravity is 1.35 g/cm^3. It was used as a tamponade for eyes with retinal detachment caused by inferior breaks.

Heavy silicone oil is also available in Europe. It is a solution of perfluorohexyloctane and silicone oil, its gravity is slightly heavier than water, and can be used for retinal detachment caused by inferior retinal breaks. The efficacy and the safety of these tamponade agents after a long follow-up are not well elucidated [21, 40].

Summary for the Clinician

- ICG staining of the ILM makes ILM peeling much easier and more complete.
- ICG is potentially toxic; however, this can be prevented or minimized by the appropriate use of ICG.
- Trypan blue (0.3%) is weaker than ICG, while it stains the proliferative membrane well.
- Triamcinolone acetonide is currently used to visualize the vitreous during vitrectomy, especially in highly myopic eyes.
- Microplasmin helps separate the vitreous hyaloid from the ILM surface.

References

1. Abrams GW, Edelhauser HF, Aaberg TM, et al. (1974) Dynamics of intravitreal sulfur hexafluoride gas. Invest Ophthalmol 13:863–868.

2. Ando F, Sasano K, Suzuki, et al. (2004) Indocyanine green-assisted ILM peeling in macular hole surgery revisited. Am J Ophthalmol 138:886–887.

3. Asami T, Terasaki H, Kachi S, et al. (2004) Ultrastructure of internal limiting membrane removed during plasmin-assisted vitrectomy from eyes with diabetic macular edema. Ophthalmology 111:231–237.

4. Brooks-HL (1995) ILM peeling in full thickness macular hole surgery. Vitreoretinal Surg Technol 7:2

5. Burk SE, Da Mata AP, Snyder ME, et al. (2000) Indocyanine green-assisted peeling of the retinal internal limiting membrane. Ophthalmology 107:2010–2014.

6. Chang S. (1987) Low viscosity liquid fluorochemicals in vitreous surgery. Am J Ophthalmol. 103:38–43.

7. Charles S. (1977) Fluid-gas exchange in the vitreous cavity. Ocutome/Fragmatome Newsletter 2:1

8. Coll GE, Change S, Sun J, et al. (1995) Perfluorocarbon liquid in the management of retinal detachment with proliferative vitreoretinopathy. Ophthalmology 102:630–638.

9. Da Mata AP, Burk SE, Foster RE, et al. (2004) Long-term follow-up of indocyanine green-assisted peeling of the retinal internal limiting membrane during vitrectomy surgery for idiopathic macular hole repair. Ophthalmology 111:2246–2253.

10. Eckardt C. (2005)Transconjunctival sutureless 23-gauge vitrectomy. Retina 25:208–211.

11. Engelbrecht NE, Freeman J, Sternberg P Jr, et al. (2002) Retinal pigment epithelial changes after macular hole surgery with indocyanine green-assisted internal limiting membrane peeling. Am J Ophthalmol 133:89–94.

12. Feron EJ, Veckeneer M, Parys-Van Ginderdeuren R, et al. (2002) Trypan blue staining of epiretinal membranes in proliferative vitreoretinopathy. Arch Ophthalmol 120:141–144.

13. Fleischman JA, Schwartz M, Dixon JA. (1981) Argon laser photocoagulation. An intraoperative trans-pars plana technique. Arch Ophthalmol 99:1610–1612.

14. Fujii GY, de Juan E, Humayun MS, et al. (2002) A new 25-gauge instrument system for transconjunctival sutureless vitrectomy surgery. Ophthalmology 109:1807–1813.

15. Fujii GY, de Juan E, Humayun MS, et al. (2002) Initial experience using the transconjunctival sutureless vitrectomy system for vitreoretinal surgery. Ophthalmology 109:1814–1820.

16. Haritoglou C, Gandorfer A, Gass CA, et al. (2002) Indocyanine green-assisted peeling of the internal limiting membrane in macular hole surgery affects visual outcome: a clinicopathologic correlation. Am J Ophthalmol 134:836–841.

17. Horiguchi M, Kojima Y, Shima Y. (2003) Removal of lens material dropped into the vitreous cavity during cataract surgery using an optical fiber-free intravitreal surgery system. J Cataract Refract Surg 29:1256–1259.

18. Kadonosono K, Itoh N, Uchio E, Nakamura S, Ohno S. (2000) Staining of internal limiting membrane in macular hole surgery. Arch Ophthalmol 118:1116–1118.

19. Kanda S, Uemura A, Yamashita T, et al. (2004) Visual field defects after intravitreous administration of indocyanine green in macular hole surgery. Arch Ophthalmol 122:1447–1451.

20. Kimura H, Kuroda S, Nagata M. (2004) Triamcinolone acetonide-assisted peeling of the internal limiting membrane. Am J Ophthalmol 137:172–173.

21. Kirchhof B, Wong D, VanMeurs J, et al. (2002) Use of perfluorohexyloctane as a long-term internal tamponade agent in complicated retinal detachment surgery. Am J Ophthalmol 133:95–101.

22. Kwok AK, Lai TY, Man-Chan W, Woo DC. (2003) Indocyanine green assisted retinal internal limiting membrane removal in stage 3 or 4 macular hole surgery. Br J Ophthalmol 87:71–74.

23. Lakhanpal RR, Humayun MS, de Juan E. (2005) Outcomes of 140 consecutive cases of 25-gauge transconjunctival surgery for posterior segment disease. Ophthalmology. 112:817–824

24. Li K, Wong D, Hiscott P, et al. (2003) Trypan blue staining of internal limiting membrane and epiretinal membrane during vitrectomy: visual results and histopathological findings. Br J Ophthalmol 87:216–219.

25. Machemer R, Steinhorst UH. (1993) Retinal separation, retinotomy, and macular relocation. II. A surgical approach for age-related macular degeneration? Graefes Arch Clin Exp Ophthalmol 231:635–641.

26. Machemer R, Buettner H, Norton EW. (1971) Vitrectomy: a pars plana approach. Trans Am Acad Ophthalmol Otolaryngol 75:813–820.

27. Margherio AR, Margherio RR, Hartzer M, et al. (1998) Plasmin enzyme-assisted vitrectomy in traumatic pediatric macular holes. Ophthalmology 105:1617–1620.

28. Nakata K, Ohji M, Ikuno Y, et al. (2004) Wide-angle viewing lens for vitrectomy. Am J Ophthalmol 137:760–762.

29. Ohji M. (2003) Retina Subspecialty Days, 2003 Annual Meeting of American Academy of Ophthalmology.

30. Ohji M, Sakaguchi H, Tano Y. (2006) Forceps with scale marks for transconjunctival sutureless vitrectomy system. Retina 26:583–585.

31. O'Malley C, Heintz RM. (1972) Vitrectomy via the pars plana—a new instrument system. Trans Pac Coast Otoophthalmol Soc Annu Meet 53:121–137.

32. Petersen J. (1987) The physical and surgical aspects of silicone oil in the vitreous cavity. Graefes Arch Clin Exp Ophthalmol 225:452–456.

33. Peyman GA, Cheema R, Conway MD et al. (2000) Triamcinolone acetonide as an aid to visualization of the vitreous and the posterior hyaloid during pars plana vitrectomy. Retina 20:554–555.

34. Sakamoto T, Miyazaki M, Hisatomi T, et al. (2002) Triamcinolone-assisted pars plana vitrectomy improves the surgical procedures and decreases the postoperative blood-ocular barrier breakdown. Graefes Arch Clin Exp Ophthalmol 240:423–429.

35. Sakuma T, Tanaka M, Mizota A, et al. (2005) Safety of in vivo pharmacologic vitreolysis with recombinant microplasmin in rabbit eyes. Invest Ophthalmol Vis Sci 46:3295–3299.

36. Sheidow TG, Blinder KJ, Holekamp N, et al. (2003) Outcome results in macular hole surgery: an evaluation of internal limiting membrane peeling with and without indocyanine green. Ophthalmology 110:1697–1701.

37. Spitznas M. (1987) A binocular indirect ophthalmomicroscope (BIOM) for non-contact wide-angle vitreous surgery. Graefes Arch Clin Exp Ophthalmol 225:13–15.

38. Williams JG, Treese MT, Williams GA, et al. (2001) Autologous plasmin enzyme in the surgical management of diabetic retinopathy. Ophthalmology 108:1902–1905.

39. Wolf S, Reichel MB, Wiedemann P, Schnurrbusch UE. (2003) Clinical findings in macular hole surgery with indocyanine green-assisted peeling of the internal limiting membrane. Graefes Arch Clin Exp Ophthalmol 241:589–592.

40. Wong D. (2005) Management of heavy silicone oil. Retina subspecialty days, 2006 Annual Meeting of American Academy of Ophthalmology, pp 162–163.

7

Chapter 8

25-Gauge Biopsy of Uveal Tumors

8

Bertil Damato, Carl Groenewald

Core Messages

- There are many different uveal tumors, not all of which are diagnosed clinically.
- Current biopsy techniques include fine-needle aspiration biopsy, trans-scleral incisional biopsy, biopsy using a 20-gauge vitreous cutter, and trans-retinal incisional biopsy.
- Trans-conjunctival, sutureless biopsy with the 25-gauge system is relatively quick and simple, and it also produces a large sample.
- The main complication is hemorrhage, which usually resolves spontaneously.
- An inadequate specimen can occur if the tumor is small and located close to the fovea, the reason for failure being the surgeon's reluctance to take a large sample, for fear of causing visual loss.
- The main indications are: diagnosis of metastasis; differentiation of melanoma from metastasis or nevus; confirmation of suspected recurrent melanoma after conservative therapy; confirmation and typing of lymphoma; and grading of a uveal melanoma.

8.1 Introduction

Uveal tumor biopsy has a long history, but is still controversial because of fears of disseminating the tumor within the eye and systemically. The recent development of the 25-gauge vitrectomy technique has increased the scope of tumor biopsy, especially in view of concurrent advances in molecular biology.

8.1.1 Uveal Tumors

There is a wide variety of uveal tumors, most of which can present with diverse clinical manifestations (Table 8.1). The most common are nevi, melanomas, and metastases, which together constitute the large majority of tumors. The remaining types are all relatively rare.

8.2 Diagnosis of Choroidal Tumors

8.2.1 Ophthalmoscopy

The large majority of choroidal tumors can readily be diagnosed on the basis of their ophthalmoscopic or slit-lamp appearances [1]. Choroidal nevi tend to be small, with a thickness of less than 2 mm, with or without drusen, and with minimal or no serous retinal detachment or lipofuscin pigment ('orange pigment'). Choroidal melanomas are usually, but not always, more than 2 mm in height, with orange pigment and serous retinal detachment, and, if Bruch's membrane is ruptured, a mushroom shape. Rarely, choroidal melanomas are diffuse. Metastases usually originate in the breast or lung, the latter possibly arising from an occult primary lesion. These tumors are characteristically amelanotic and rapid-growing, with indistinct margins and a marked exudative retinal detachment. Choroidal hemangiomas are usually pink, with or without exudative retinal detachment, and almost all are located far posteriorly.

Table 8.1 Uveal tumors classified according to pathogenesis and location [28]. *RPE* retinal pigment epithelium

Category	Subtype		Location		
			Iris	Ciliary body	Choroid
Inflammatory	Infectious	Granuloma	+	+	+
	Non-infectious	Sarcoidosis	+	+	+
		Juvenile xanthogranuloma	+	+	
		Scleritis		+	+
		Uveal effusion		+	+
Neoplastic/hamartomatous					
Benign	Melanocytes				
		Melanocytic nevus	+	+	+
		Melanocytosis	+	+	+
		Melanocytoma	+	+	+
		Lisch nodules	+		
		Bilateral diffuse uveal melanocytic hyperplasia		+	+
	Epithelium	Cyst	+	+	
		RPE detachment			+
		Reactive epithelial hyperplasia		+	+
		Adenomatous hyperplasia		+	+
		Adenoma	+	+	+
		Congenital hypertrophy of RPE			+
		Medulloepithelioma		+	+
		Combined hamartoma of retina and RPE			+
	Blood vessels	Circumscribed hemangioma			+
		Diffuse hemangioma		+	+
		Hemangiopericytoma	+		+
		Racemose angioma	+		
	Fibroblasts	Neurofibroma	+	+	+
	Neural tissue	Neurilemmoma		+	+
	Muscle	Leiomyoma	+	+	+
		Mesectodermal leiomyoma	+	+	
	Lymphocytes	Lymphoid tumor	+	+	+
	Foreign	Lacrimal gland choristoma	+	+	
		Glioneuroma	+	+	

8

Table 8.1 (*continued*)

Category	Subtype		Location		
			Iris	Ciliary body	Choroid
Malignant	Melanocytes	Melanoma	+	+	+
	Epithelium	Adenocarcinoma	+	+	+
		Medulloepithelioma	+	+	+
	Muscle	Rhabdo/leiomyosarcoma	+	+	
	Secondary	Melanoma/carcinoma	+	+	+
	Hemopoietic	Lymphoma	+	+	+
		Leukemia	+	+	+
	Metastatic	Carcinoma/sarcoma	+	+	+
Traumatic		Foreign body	+	+	+
		Implantation cyst	+		
		Miotic cyst	+		
		Suprachoroidal hematoma			+
Degenerative		Disciform lesion			+
		Sclerochoroidal calcification			+
Idiopathic		Osteoma			+
		Vasoproliferative tumor			+
		Varicose vortex vein			+

8.2.2 Angiography

Fluorescein angiography is not particularly helpful in distinguishing between the various choroidal tumors, being most useful for recording secondary changes, particularly after radiotherapy and other conservative therapy. Indocyanine green angiography is better at demonstrating the extent of a choroidal tumor and can provide some diagnostic clues, such as dye wash-out in choroidal hemangiomas.

8.2.3 Echography

Echography is most useful for detecting the presence of an intraocular tumor, if the media are opaque, for example because of cataract or vitreous hemorrhage. This investigation can also re-veal extraocular tumor extension. B-scan ultrasonography can demonstrate a mushroom shape, which is almost pathognomonic of melanoma. The internal acoustic reflectivity, best demonstrated by standardized A-scan echography, is helpful in diagnosis. For example, it tends to be absent with retinal pigment epithelial detachment, low with uveal melanoma, moderate with metastasis, and high with hemangioma.

8.2.4 Other Investigations

Computerized tomography and magnetic resonance imaging are used mostly for treatment planning. The P32 (radioactive phosphorus) test has become obsolete. Immunoscintigraphy is not widely performed.

8

Summary for the Clinician

- Most uveal tumors can be diagnosed by slit-lamp and ophthalmoscopic examination.
- Uveal tumor biopsy is rarely necessary.

8.3 Current Biopsy Techniques

8.3.1 Fine Needle Aspiration Biopsy

Fine needle aspiration biopsy (FNAB) is the technique that is most widely used today for sampling intraocular tumors [2]. Most use a 25-gauge needle, which is believed to be associated with a smaller risk of tumor seeding than when a larger needle is used [3]. The pars plana approach is the most favored, although some prefer to pass the needle through the sclera directly over the tumor (Fig. 8.1). The need for suction is disputed [4]. The greatest problem is an inadequate sample size, which is most likely to occur with small tumors [5]. Some regard failure to obtain sufficient material as an indication that the tumor cells are highly cohesive and therefore likely to be benign [6]. FNAB has also been used for iris tumors, with a successful result in most patients [2, 7, 8].

8.3.2 Trans-Scleral Tumor Biopsy

Trans-scleral local resection of uveal tumors is in effect an excisional biopsy, because in addition to eliminating the tumor it also provides tissue for histological diagnosis [9]. Indeed, for ciliary body tumors, diagnostication is now the primary reason for iridocyclectomy, which has been replaced by proton beam radiotherapy, in Liverpool at least (Fig. 8.2) [10]. Excisional biopsy of choroidal tumors has also been performed in a small number of patients [11].

Incisional biopsy is performed using techniques similar to those developed for trans-scleral local resection, except that the lamellar scleral flap is triangular instead of rectangular, to reduce the number of sutures required. This technique can also be used for iris tumors (Fig. 8.3). Incisional biopsy of the ciliary body and choroidal tumors produces a larger sample than FNAB, but is a relatively long procedure requiring moderate systemic hypotension to reduce hemorrhage. Orbital tumor recurrence has been reported after trans-scleral incisional biopsy [2]. This procedure is therefore contraindicated for posterior tumors unless immediate brachytherapy is delivered, the duration of plaque insertion being determined by the result of the biopsy.

8.3.3 20-Gauge Vitreous Cutter

The 20-gauge vitreous cutter has been used to biopsy both iris and choroidal tumors, the latter involving three-port vitrectomy and gas tamponade [12]. This method produced a larger sample than FNAB and avoided the risks of orbital seeding that are associated with trans-scleral incisional biopsy.

8.3.4 Trans-Vitreal Incisional Biopsy

Recently, Kvanta and associates described pars plana vitrectomy-assisted incisional biopsy, removing the sample with intraocular forceps and a diamond knife; however, they reported significant ocular complications [13].

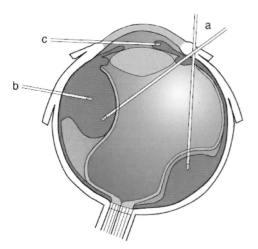

Fig. 8.1 Approaches for fine-needle aspiration biopsy. *a* Trans-vitreal for choroidal and ciliary body tumors; *b* trans-scleral for ciliary body or choroidal tumors, prior to brachytherapy; *c* trans-corneal for anterior chamber tumors

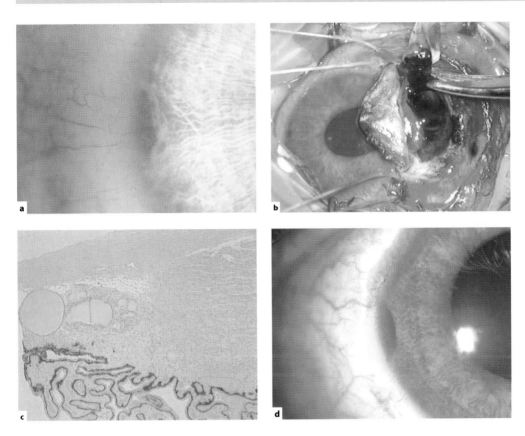

Fig. 8.2   Excision biopsy of a multicystic iridociliary tumor in the right eye of a 15-year-old male. **a** Preoperative appearance. **b** Intraoperative photograph. **c** Light micrograph, showing thyroid tissue. **d** Postoperative appearance, when the vision had improved to 6/6. A diagnosis of ectopic thyroid was made, based on negative systemic findings, even after prolonged follow-up [10]

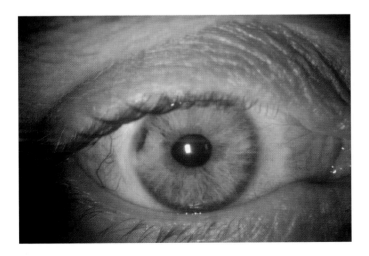

Fig. 8.3   Incisional biopsy of an iris tumor in a 31-year-old female, which proved to be an amelanotic melanoma of spindle-B type. The patient was treated with proton beam radiotherapy. Almost 5 years later, the vision was 6/6 with no complications

8

8.3.5 25-Gauge Biopsy Technique

When trans-conjunctival, sutureless vitrectomy using the 25-G system was first described, we were impressed by the convenience and simplicity of this approach [14]. In 2004, we started using this system for intraocular tumor biopsy, because we felt that this method would provide a better sample than FNAB and that it would be quicker and safer than trans-scleral incisional biopsy and trans-vitreal biopsy using the 20-gauge vitreous cutter. To date, we have performed about 40 procedures using the 25-gauge system, which has become established as our preferred technique. When we started performing intraocular tumor biopsy with the 25-gauge vitreous cutter we were not aware of any previous biopsy experience with this system, although Finger et al. have since reported using such equipment for biopsy of iris lesions [15].

8.4 Preoperative Management

The patient is assessed in the conventional manner, taking a full history, examining both eyes, performing ocular ultrasonography, and undertaking other ocular and systemic investigations selectively. Informed consent is obtained in the usual fashion, recording all risks by completing a standard form in the patient's charts. An audio cassette tape recording of the discussion is given to all patients to help them remember what was said.

8.5 Surgical Technique

The procedure is performed under local anesthesia, with a retrobulbar block. The infusion port, light pipe, and vitreous cutter are inserted 3.5 mm from the limbus. To separate the conjunctival and scleral openings, the conjunctiva is pulled parallel to the sclera with nontoothed forceps during insertion of the trochar for the microcannula. If tantalum markers or a radioactive plaque is inserted during the same operation, the tumor biopsy is performed after these procedures are completed, with the ports passed through undisturbed conjunctiva. The vitreous cutter is advanced across the vitreous cavity and through the retina into the center of the tumor. Tissue samples are taken by rotating the cutter within the tumor. The vitreous cutter is withdrawn from the tumor to flush the aspiration line if tumor tissue blocks the cutter. Total vitrectomy is not performed so as to allow contact between the vitreous base and the retinal opening. Suction is stopped before the aspirate reaches the three-way tap and the cutter is removed from the vitreous. The specimen is back-flushed into a gallipot through the cutter. With the operating microscope, tumor fragments are visible in the gallipot, confirming that an adequate sample has been obtained. When the microcannulae are removed a cotton bud is used to ensure separation of the conjunctival and scleral openings. Gas tamponade is not used. The aspirate is placed in a sterile container with an equal volume of 10% neutral buffered formalin.

8.6 Care of Specimen

In the laboratory, this preparation is then centrifuged. The resulting pellet is embedded in agar and the preparation was processed into paraffin wax. Sections of the resulting wax-embedded cell block were stained by hematoxylin and eosin, the periodic acid Schiff technique or immunohistochemical methods, as previously described.

8.7 Postoperative Management

All patients are re-examined on the first postoperative day and then within 7 days of surgery at our center or by the referring ophthalmologist. Topical antibiotic, steroid, and cycloplegic drops are administered in the standard fashion as for other vitrectomy procedures.

In patients in whom a ruthenium plaque is applied, the radiation doses required for both melanoma and metastasis are calculated. Once the histopathological diagnosis is known, 1 or 2 days after the plaque insertion, arrangements are made to remove the plaque as soon as the appropriate dose of radiation has been delivered.

Summary for the Clinician

- Trans-conjunctival, sutureless, 25-gauge biopsy of posterior segment tumors is performed using three ports, for infusion, illumination, and the vitrector.
- Retinopexy and gas tamponade are not required.
- Anterior segment biopsy is performed through a clear cornea.
- Insertion of a radioactive plaque or tantalum markers for proton beam radiotherapy should be performed before the biopsy.

8.8 Results and Complications

8.8.1 Adequacy of Sample

In most patients, the sample size is much greater than that previously obtained with FNAB [16]. The larger specimen facilitates immunohistochemistry using multiple antibodies (Fig. 8.4) and there is usually sufficient tissue for cytogenetic studies to be undertaken (Fig. 8.5). An inadequate sample occasionally occurs, mostly if the procedure is deliberately curtailed because the tumor is small and located close to the fovea. The larger yield provided by the 25-gauge system compared with FNAB and the ability to see tumor fragments in a gallipot held under the operating microscope have reduced the need for a pathologist to be present in the operating theater at the time of the biopsy.

8.8.2 Sampling Error

When biopsy is performed to grade a melanoma, there is a possibility that the tumor is heterogeneous, in which case the lack of adverse histological or cytogenetic findings might be the result of a sampling error. The chances of such an error occurring would be reduced by taking biopsies from several different sites; if the tumor is large; however, this may increase the risk of complications.

8.8.3 Tumor Seeding

With malignant neoplasms, there is a risk of seeding viable tumor cells to other parts of the eye and to the sclerotomy sites. With metastases to the eye, this should not be a problem, because the whole eye is irradiated in such cases. With melanoma, however, seeding may cause recurrences both within the eye and extraocularly. Experience with FNAB suggests that these risks are extremely small, probably because few melanomas have the capacity to seed to retina. With the 25-gauge vitrectomy system, the cannulae should further diminish any possibility of seeding to the sclerotomy sites, when choroidal tumors are biopsied. With iris tumors, there is perhaps a greater theoretical risk of spreading tumor to iris and trabecular meshwork, which, unlike the choroid and ciliary body, are not covered by neural tissue. However, most iris melanomas are low-grade and therefore unlikely to seed readily whereas the minority of iris melanomas that are aggressive have probably already spread diffusely and seeded around the anterior chamber by the time the patient first presents.

8.8.4 Hemorrhage

Hemorrhage is the most common complication of tumor biopsy performed with the 25-gauge vitreous cutter. Usually the hemorrhage is mild and resolves spontaneously after a few days (Fig. 8.4n). Subretinal hemorrhage can occur and in one of our patients involved the fovea (Fig. 8.5c). Our impression is that hemorrhage is more severe when the tumor is small, possibly because damage to normal choroidal vessels is more likely in such cases. It is also possible that in some patients hemorrhage is induced or aggravated by postoperative hypotony, which can occur in a minority of patients as a result of fluid leakage through the unsutured sclerotomy.

The reasons why, in combined procedures, biopsy is performed after insertion of a radioactive plaque or tantalum markers, and not before, are (1) so that any immediate hemorrhage caused by the biopsy will not complicate the plaque or marker insertion, by hindering tumor localiza-

8

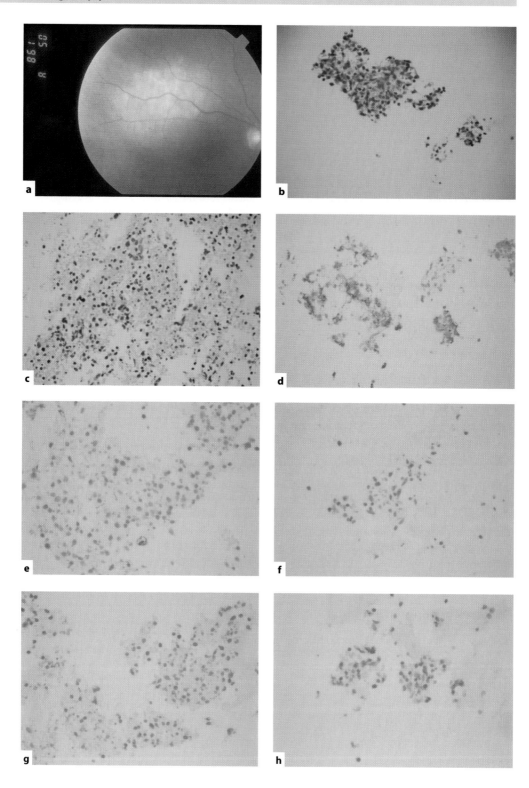

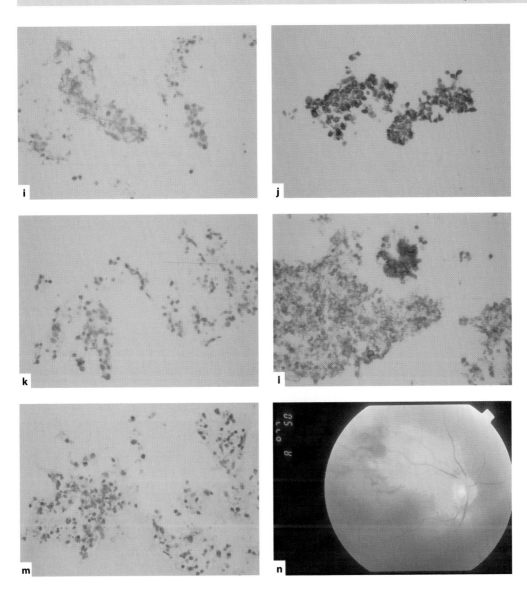

Fig. 8.4 The 25-gauge biopsy of suspected choroidal metastasis in the right eye of a 69-year-old man. **a** Preoperative photograph showing an amelanotic tumor, which measured 11.2 × 9.8 × 2.7 mm on ultrasonography. **b** Hematoxylin and eosin, showing malignant cells. **c** Hematoxylin and eosin, showing necrotic tissue. **d** Keratin stain (positive). **e** Melan-A stain for melanocytes (negative). **f** HMB-45 stain for melanoma (negative). **g** Prostate-specific antigen (negative). **h** Prostatic alkaline phosphatase (negative). **i** Cytokeratin antigen (negative). **j** CK8/18 antigen for glandular cells (positive). **k** CK7 for ductal cells (negative). **l** CD56 antigen for ectodermal neural cells (positive), and **m** CD45 for leukocytes (negative). **n** Early postoperative photograph showing mild hemorrhage, which resolved spontaneously. Additional specimens were available for cytogenetic studies, in case the tumor had proved to be a melanoma. The primary tumor was identified as a neuroendocrine carcinoma, probably arising in the lung

8

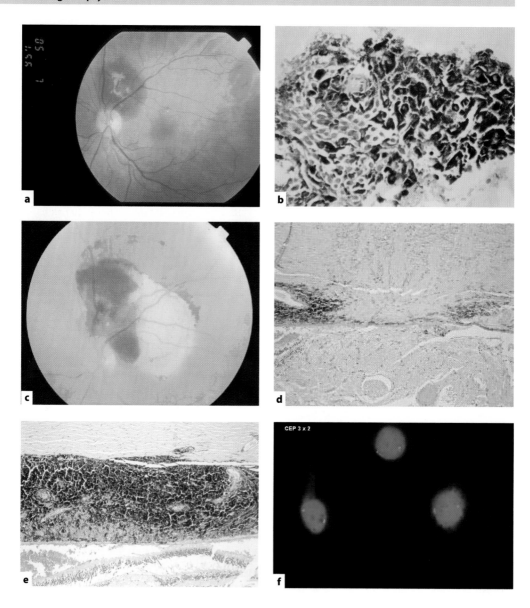

Fig. 8.5 Juxtapapillary choroidal tumor, measuring 4.5 × 3.8 × 1.5 mm, in the left eye of a 71-year-old man. The differential diagnosis included nevus and melanoma. **a** The tumor showed surface orange pigment, which suggested the latter diagnosis despite the small tumor size. **b** The patient requested biopsy so that the eye would be removed if the tumor was proven to be malignant. Biopsy confirmed that the tumor was a malignant melanoma of spindle-B cell type. **c** Postoperatively a sub-retinal hemorrhage was present, which extended to the fovea. **d** Histological examination of the enucleated eye showed the tumor to be more extensive than pre-operative assessment had indicated, completely encircling the optic disk and **e** there was deep scleral invasion. Cytogenetic studies showed no evidence of monosomy 3. If the patient had been observed for growth, the tumor may have had time to extend extraocularly. Treatment with transpupillary thermotherapy would have failed because it would have been administered only to the visible tumor superior to the optic disk. Radiotherapy would probably have caused severe visual loss and perhaps painful neovascular complications. It is not known whether the tumor would have developed monosomy 3 and metastasized if left untreated

tion and (2) so that ocular hypotony and hemorrhage will not be caused by the surgical manipulations required for the implant insertion.

8.8.5 Rhegmatogenous Retinal Detachment

We have not seen rhegmatogenous retinal detachment in any of our patients, despite omitting retinopexy and internal tamponade (although one of our patients was treated surgically for retinal detachment by the referring ophthalmologist despite our reassurance that this was exudative and not rhegmatogenous). Our encouraging experience is similar to that of trans-retinal FNAB, which is generally performed without laser treatment or intraocular gas injection. Our impression is that the tumor itself and any associated exudation tamponade the retinotomy.

8.8.6 Other Complications

Other potential complications are the same as for other vitrectomy procedures using the 25-gauge system and include: iatrogenic retinal breaks; inadvertently touching the lens; endophthalmitis; postoperative ocular hypertension; postoperative hypotony; and intraoperative breakage of the 25-gauge vitreous cutter [17].

Summary for the Clinician

- The most frequent complication is hemorrhage, which is usually mild.
- An inadequate specimen can result, especially from small tumors.

8.9 Indications and Contraindications

8.9.1 Indications

8.9.1.1 Diagnosis of Metastasis

In our clinic, the commonest indication for choroidal tumor biopsy is to determine the site of the primary malignancy in a patient with an unequivocal metastasis. This information facilitates subsequent management by an oncologist, for example, by directing investigation to particular organs (Fig. 8.4).

8.9.1.2 Differentiation Between Metastasis and Melanoma

Rarely, tumor biopsy is indicated to confirm a clinical diagnosis of melanoma or metastasis. For example, a patient with a lightly pigmented tumor has a past history of malignancy, casting doubt on the likely diagnosis of amelanotic melanoma. Some indistinct amelanotic tumors have features consistent with both melanoma and metastasis, making histological studies a necessity (Fig. 8.6)

8.9.1.3 Differentiation Between Nevus and Melanoma

Melanocytic tumors of indeterminate malignancy are not unusual in a specialist ocular oncology service such as ours (Fig. 8.5). The standard practice is to observe such lesions until growth is documented by photography, ultrasonography, or both [18]. Such delayed treatment can be considered safe only if it is assumed that uveal melanomas start to metastasize after they have grown large. There is growing circumstantial evidence, based on estimated tumor doubling times, that metastatic spread begins early, several years before treatment, and when tumors are very small, possibly less than 2 mm in diameter [19, 20]. According to this hypothesis, it is the small melanomas that should be treated most urgently because it is with these tumors that any opportunities for

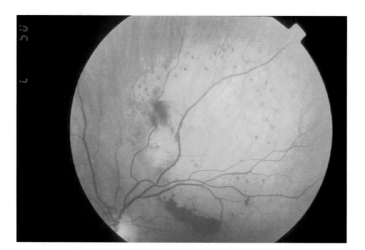

Fig. 8.6 Amelanotic choroidal tumor in the left eye of a 56-year-old woman. The tumor measured 10.5 × 10.0 × 1.6 mm. The differential diagnosis included amelanotic nevus, melanoma, and metastasis. Biopsy confirmed the diagnosis of melanoma and the patient underwent proton beam radiotherapy. The figure shows the fundus appearance shortly after biopsy, with a small hemorrhage of no significance

preventing metastatic spread are greatest. Biopsy, therefore, seems a reasonable alternative to prolonged observation in such cases [6]. Unfortunately, these are the tumors that are most difficult to sample, whatever technique is used.

8.9.1.4　Confirmation of Local Recurrence of Melanoma after Conservative Treatment

After radiotherapy, tumor enlargement does not necessarily indicate malignant growth. The first author has performed endo-resection on a few patients whose enlarging tumor after radiotherapy proved to consist of macrophages (Fig. 8.7). In such cases, there would be scope for performing a biopsy if enucleation is being considered.

8.9.1.5　Confirmation of Intraocular Lymphoma

In view of the rarity of intraocular lymphomas, it is conventional to confirm the diagnosis by means of biopsy (Fig. 8.8). This is especially the case with suspected uveal lymphocytic proliferations (Fig. 8.9).

8.9.1.6　Prognosis

Choroidal and ciliary melanomas tend to develop partial or complete loss of chromosome 3 (i.e., monosomy 3) [21, 22]. In addition, they tend to show gains of the long arm of chromosome 8 [21, 22]. They also develop gains in the short arm of chromosome 6 [23]. Monosomy 3 is associated with a reduction in the actuarial 5-year survival probability from over 90% to less than 50% [24, 25]. Chromosome 8 gains are also associated with an adverse prognosis. Conversely, gains in chromosome 6p indicate a very good chance of survival [23]. It has been suggested that monosomy 3 and disomy 3 melanomas represent two separate classes of melanoma, which are totally distinct from their initiation [26]. We and others have found uveal melanomas containing both monosomy 3 and disomy 3 melanoma cells, which suggests that low-grade, disomy 3 melanomas transform into the high-grade monosomy 3 variety. About 30% of small melanomas (i.e., about 10 mm in diameter) are of the high-grade variety compared with about 50% of large tumors [25]. It is uncertain whether transformation from low-grade to high-grade occurs in large tumors, if treatment is delayed, or whether large tumor size is merely an indicator of increased malignancy, with high-grade tumors tending to be larger at the time of treatment because they grow more rapidly. In any case, cytogenetics seems to be superior to largest basal tumor diameter, tumor

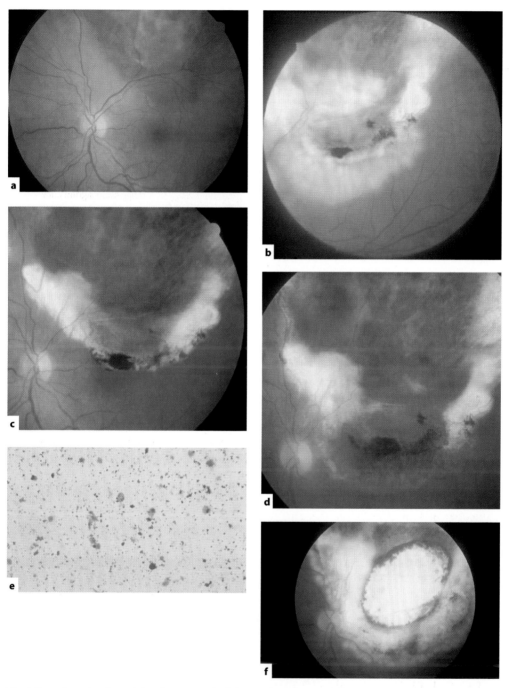

Fig. 8.7 **a** Superior choroidal melanoma in the left eye of a 34-year-old woman, who was treated by the first author with ruthenium plaque brachytherapy in May 1988. **b** Tumor recurrence developed at the inferior margin, which was treated with photocoagulation. **c, d** Despite repeated phototherapy, the tumor grew progressively. **e** In August 1993, the recurrent tumor was removed by endo-resection and was found to consist of melanomacrophages, with no evidence of any viable tumor. **f** One month postoperatively, the eye settled well, without complications. Sixteen years postoperatively, the patient was healthy, with no sign of local or systemic recurrence and she was able to count fingers, with a useful temporal field

8

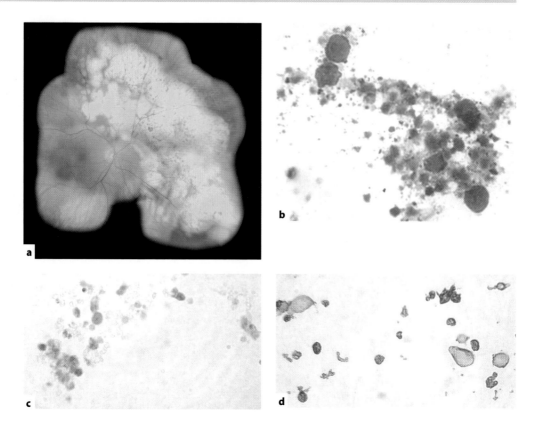

Fig. 8.8 Suspected lymphoma in the right eye of a 72-year-old woman. **a** Fundus appearance. **b** Giemsa stain, showing large malignant cells consistent with lymphoma. **c** CD3 stain for T lymphocytes (negative). **d** CD20 stain for B lymphocytes (positive)

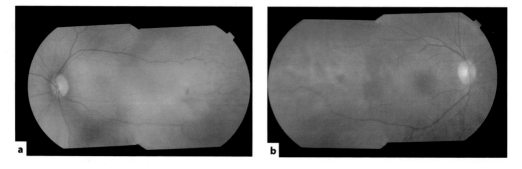

Fig. 8.9 Uveal lymphoma in the left eye of a 72-year-old woman. **a** Left fundus, 5 months after 25-gauge biopsy, showing a small scar at the site of the retinotomy. **b** Normal right fundus. The patient was treated with external beam radiotherapy

cell type, extravascular matrix patterns and other prognostic indicators when estimating the probability of metastatic disease [25].

There seems to be much scope for determining whether a choroidal melanoma is low-grade or high-grade. First, if a small melanoma is found to be high-grade, and therefore life-threatening, it is likely that treatment would be administered without delay, in the hope that metastatic spread has not yet occurred, and any iatrogenic ocular morbidity would be more acceptable. Second, a small, high-grade melanoma is more likely to be treated with radiotherapy or enucleation than by transpupillary thermotherapy. This is because such treatment is associated with a three-year recurrence rate of 22% [27]. It is noteworthy that this incidence of recurrence is similar to the prevalence of monosomy 3 in small tumors, in the authors' series. Third, determination of the grade of melanoma malignancy profoundly influences patient care, individuals with a disomy 3 melanoma being greatly reassured of their relatively good prognosis, whereas those with a high-grade tumor are referred to an oncologist for consideration of regular screening for systemic metastases. Hopefully, it will soon be possible for patients with a poor prognosis to be entered into randomized, prospective studies of systemic adjuvant therapy. The scope of 25-gauge biopsy will increase if such adjuvant therapy were to become available.

The apparent lack of monosomy 3 in a biopsy specimen does not necessarily guarantee a good prognosis. First, a sampling error can occur in a heterogeneous tumor. Second, a lethal partial deletion may be missed if this is small. Third, it is not known at what stage transformation from low-grade to high-grade melanoma becomes unlikely. For example, it is uncertain whether a chromosome 6 abnormality indicates that monosomy 3 is unlikely to develop.

Biopsy is also of prognostic value for other diseases, such as lymphoproliferative tumors.

8.9.2 Contraindications

The main contraindication to intraocular tumor biopsy is retinoblastoma, because of the high probability of tumor seeding into extraocular

tissues. The risks associated with biopsy of other tumors, such as medulloepithelioma and adenocarcinoma, are essentially unknown.

Summary for the Clinician

- The main indications are:
  - Diagnosis of metastasis.
  - Differentiation between metastasis and melanoma.
  - Differentiation between nevus and melanoma.
  - Confirmation of diagnosis of recurrent melanoma after radiotherapy.
  - Confirmation of diagnosis and characterization of lymphoma.
  - Grading of uveal melanoma.

8.10 Conclusions

Although no randomized, prospective studies have been performed, evidence suggests that in general uveal tumor biopsy with the 25-gauge vitreous cutter produces a larger sample than FNAB and more quickly and safely than transscleral incisional biopsy or using the 20-gauge vitrectomy system. Early results are encouraging, but it is likely that results will improve with further refinements of the technique and developments in laboratory methods.

References

1. Damato B. *Ocular tumours: Diagnosis and Treatment*. Oxford: Butterworth Heinemann, 2000, pp 57–93.
2. Char DH, Kemlitz AE, Miller T. Intraocular biopsy. *Ophthalmol. Clin. North Am.* 2005;**18**:177–185.
3. Glasgow BJ, Brown HH, Zargoza AM, *et al.* Quantitation of tumor seeding from fine needle aspiration of ocular melanomas. *Am. J. Ophthalmol.* 1988;**105**:538–546.
4. Midena E, Segato T, Piermarocchi S, *et al.* Fine needle aspiration biopsy in ophthalmology. *Surv. Ophthalmol.* 1985;**29**:410–422.

5. Cohen VM, Dinakaran S, Parsons MA, *et al.* Transvitreal fine needle aspiration biopsy: the influence of intraocular lesion size on diagnostic biopsy result. *Eye* 2001;**15**:143–147.

6. Augsburger JJ, Correa ZM, Schneider S, *et al.* Diagnostic transvitreal fine-needle aspiration biopsy of small melanocytic choroidal tumors in nevus versus melanoma category. *Trans. Am. Ophthalmol. Soc.* 2002;**100**:225–232; discussion 232–234.

7. Shields JA, Shields CL, Ehya H, *et al.* Fine-needle aspiration biopsy of suspected intraocular tumors. The 1992 Urwick Lecture. *Ophthalmology* 1993;**100**:1677–1684.

8. Grossniklaus HE. Fine-needle aspiration biopsy of the iris. *Arch. Ophthalmol.* 1992;**110**:969–976.

9. Damato BE, Foulds WS. In: Schachat AP, Ryan SJ, eds. *Retina.* 4th ed. St Louis: Mosby, 2006:769–778.

10. Tiberti A, Damato B, Hiscott P, Vora J. Iris ectopic thyroid tissue. Report of a case. Arch. Ophthalmol. 2006 (in press).

11. Brannan SO, Lessan NG, Hiscott P, *et al.* A choroidal amyloid-rich neuroendocrine tumor: initial manifestation of Cushing syndrome. *Arch. Ophthalmol.* 1999;**117**:1081–1083.

12. Bechrakis NE, Foerster MH, Bornfeld N. Biopsy in indeterminate intraocular tumors. *Ophthalmology* 2002;**109**:235–242.

13. Kvanta A, Seregard S, Kopp ED, *et al.* Choroidal biopsies for intraocular tumors of indeterminate origin. *Am. J. Ophthalmol.* 2005;**140**:1002–1006.

14. Fujii GY, De Juan E Jr, Humayun MS, *et al.* A new 25-gauge instrument system for transconjunctival sutureless vitrectomy surgery. *Ophthalmology* 2002;**109**:1807–1812.

15. Finger PT, Latkany P, Kurli M *et al.* The Finger iridectomy technique: small incision biopsy of anterior segment tumours. *Br. J. Ophthalmol.* 2005;**89**:946–949.

16. Sen J, Groenewald C, Hiscott PS, Smith P, Damato BE. Trans-retinal choroidal tumor biopsy with a 25-gauge vitrector. *Ophthalmology* 2006;**113**:1028–1031.

17. Inoue M, Noda K, Ishida S, *et al.* Intraoperative breakage of a 25-gauge vitreous cutter. *Am. J. Ophthalmol.* 2004;**138**:867–869.

18. Collaborative Ocular Melanoma Study Group. Factors predictive of growth and treatment of small choroidal melanoma. COMS report no. 5. *Arch. Ophthalmol.* 1997;**115**:1537–1544.

19. Manschot WA, Lee WR, van Strik R. Uveal melanoma: updated considerations on current management modalities. *Int. Ophthalmol.* 1995;**19**:203–209.

20. Eskelin S, Pyrhonen S, Summanen P, *et al.* Tumor doubling times in metastatic malignant melanoma of the uvea: tumor progression before and after treatment. *Ophthalmology* 2000;**107**:1443–1449.

21. Horsman DE, Sroka H, Rootman J, *et al.* Monosomy 3 and isochromosome 8q in a uveal melanoma. *Cancer Genet. Cytogenet.* 1990;**45**:249–253.

22. Horsthemke B, Prescher G, Bornfeld N, *et al.* Loss of chromosome 3 alleles and multiplication of chromosome 8 alleles in uveal melanoma. *Genes Chromosomes Cancer* 1992;**4**:217–221.

23. Parrella P, Sidransky D, Merbs SL. Allelotype of posterior uveal melanoma: implications for a bifurcated tumor progression pathway. *Cancer Res.* 1999;**59**:3032–3037.

24. Prescher G, Bornfeld N, Hirche H, *et al.* Prognostic implications of monosomy 3 in uveal melanoma. *Lancet* 1996;**347**:1222–1225.

25. Scholes AG, Damato BE, Nunn J, *et al.* Monosomy 3 in uveal melanoma: correlation with clinical and histologic predictors of survival. *Invest. Ophthalmol. Vis. Sci.* 2003;**44**:1008–1011.

26. Tschentscher F, Husing J, Holter T, *et al.* Tumor classification based on gene expression profiling shows that uveal melanomas with and without monosomy 3 represent two distinct entities. *Cancer Res.* 2003;**63**:2578–2584.

27. Shields CL, Shields JA, Perez N, *et al.* Primary transpupillary thermotherapy for small choroidal melanoma in 256 consecutive cases: outcomes and limitations. *Ophthalmology* 2002;**109**:225–234.

28. Damato B, Coupland S, Hiscott PS. Classification of uveal tumors. In: Clinical ocular oncology, Eds. Singh AD, Damato BE, Pe-er J, Murphree AL, Perry JD. Elsevier, Amsterdam (in press).

8

Chapter 9

Vitrectomy Against Floaters

9

Hans Hoerauf

Core Messages

- Despite minimal objective findings vitreous opacities can produce severe psychological strain.
- The risk of complications of vitrectomy in patients with mouches volantes seems to be low.
- Patient selection is more time consuming than in many other ocular pathologies, but guarantees the likelihood of subjective postoperative success.
- In the evaluation of individual factors, a longer and more thorough history is neccessary.
- Severe vision-impairing complications will occur in an increasing number of patients.
- Visual acuity testing alone cannot account for the disabling symptoms and is not an adequate parameter for the indication of vitrectomy in this group of patients. Difficulties in daily life caused by opacification may be more relevant inclusion criteria.
- Better tests are urgently required to assist in the detailed analysis and grading of difficulties caused by vitreous floaters.
- It is important to rule out other possible subtle causes of the symptoms such as uveitis, corneal endothelial failure, posterior capsular opacity or cystoid macular edema.
- Despite the simple surgical technique for vitreous opacities, vitrectomy in affected patients who have a high potential for visual acuity, should be performed by an experienced vitreoretinal surgeon.

9.1 Introduction

Vitrectomy may be indicated in a selected group of patients with visually disturbing vitreous floaters, but the objective assessment of visual dysfunction from vitreous floaters is very difficult. Visual acuity testing alone cannot account for the disabling symptoms, but a too liberal indication of vitrectomy in patients with this common problem may lead to potential misuse and vitreoretinal lifestyle surgery.

In the past, the general concept of most vitreoretinal surgeons was that the better the visual function the lower the indication for an elective vitrectomy. Patients with full visual acuity and without evident ocular pathology are generally not seen as candidates for vitrectomy. This restraining and conservative logic has several reasons:

- Complications of vitrectomy were previously much more frequent and severe [15, 23];
- It is hard to believe that mouches volantes cause a reduction in the quality of life;
- Patients asking for surgery despite full visual acuity may have difficult personalities and may be more likely to complain and cause problems after surgery.

However, current vitrectomy techniques carry a markedly lower risk of complications and the treatment of complications has improved. The assumed neurotic personality of patients complaining about mouches volantes has been based on unproven prejudices and the effect of mouches volantes on quality of life has never been investigated.

In this article the author will discuss:

- Whether vitrectomy is justified in patients with full visual acuity and subjectively disturbing floaters that are objectively minimal and hardly detectable;

- Which precautions are helpful to minimize possible risks and complications;
- Which guidelines should be established when considering surgery for floaters.

9.2 Clinical Findings

Vitreous opacities, so called "floaters" or "mouches volantes" may occur in normal eyes as well as in eyes of patients with vitreoretinal disorders. In rare cases vitreous floaters may also develop after cataract extraction [4] and scleral buckling surgery. Floaters are caused by condensed vitreous fibers or glial tissue of epipapillary origin that adhere to the posterior vitreous cortex [7] and result in entoptic phenomena. Myopic patients are more likely to develop vitreous floaters [4]. Floaters may cause symptoms depending on their size, density, mobility, and proximity to the retina. A high incidence of posterior vitreous detachment (PVD) in eyes with suddenly appearing floaters has been reported [16, 14, 21] and this incidence is even higher when only patients over 50 years of age are considered. A dense opacity in the prepapillary area is an indicator of PVD. This correlates with most of the studies reporting vitrectomy for vitreous floaters in which a high incidence of PVD was described. This opacity attached to the posterior hyaloid must be differentiated from opacity in the gel associated with vitreous liquefaction.

Although PVD is often present in patients with symptomatic floaters [21], such opacities may also be intravitreal and not associated with PVD. These fiber-like intravitreal opacities appear to result from the condensation and contraction of the vitreous framework after liquefaction of the gel. Vitreous liquefaction begins at a relatively young age in patients with high myopia and progresses with age and axial elongation. A number of studies have addressed the relationship between liquefaction of the vitreous and high myopia [9, 19, 29]. It has been shown that in cases of high myopia, advanced liquefaction without PVD results in large lacuna formation [9, 29]. The lacunae become larger and confluent with advancing age. Analysis of postmortem eyes that included highly myopic eyes

in which the axial length exceeded 26 mm had shown that hyaluronic acid collagen concentrations within the vitreous were much lower in these eyes than in the emmetropic eyes [2]. This biochemical change may be related to earlier liquefaction and opacification in high myopia. In a thoroughly performed study including 148 eyes Murakami et al. described prepapillary glial tissue on the posterior hyaloid membrane and minimal vitreous hemorrhage as the primary cause of symptomatic floaters [21]. In patients without PVD, Murakami et al. observed intravitreal fiber-like opacities corresponding to the patient's symptoms in the posterior vitreous cavity near the retina. They found these opacifications on the plicated membranes of Cloque's canal, and also in association with liquefaction of the gel.

9.3 Symptoms and Natural Course

Most of the vitreous opacities are located anterior to areas of vitreous liquefaction, and are therefore far in front of the retina. Opacities may only cause symptoms if they are close to the retina in front of the posterior pole, or if they are large and dense enough. Visible vitreous opacities vary in shape, size, and density and are fibrous in appearance. Because of the extreme mobility of the gel, the appearance and location of these opacities vary considerably. Typical ring-shaped opacities are rare. Opacities are often located at the margin of the lacuna and become symptomatic when they form condensation along the visual axis. The related symptoms are multiple and vague. Only in a few cases the complaints are clearly associated with the presence of large fibrous masses. Centrovitreal location of opacities can reduce visual acuity by impeding the visual axis. However, it is important that vitreous floaters, whether secondary to posterior vitreous detachment or to syneresis and fibrillar degeneration, often become less symptomatic and troublesome with the passage of time often as the posterior hyaloid migrates anteriorly in the vitreous cavity. Furthermore, patients can become accustomed to and less aware of their floaters. After explanation and information from their ophthalmologists about the harmless nature of vitreous opacities, many patients are relieved and can live with the symptoms. However, the natural history can be variable and a minority of patients with persistent, distracting and disabling symptoms will remain. In this group of patients the perception of floaters in the visual field can cause significant visual disability. Affected patients complain that tasks requiring work at near and distance become difficult, concentration becomes impaired and productivity declines.

9.4 Diagnostic Methods

Most importantly, primary floaters have to be distinguished from secondary floaters caused by an underlying ocular pathology, such as uveitis, vitreous haemmorhage, asteroid hyalosis [22] or amyloidosis. Conventional techniques of vitreous biomicroscopy make it difficult to detect subtle changes in the vitreous and vitreoretinal relationships. When a PVD is present, jerky ocular movements momentarily displace the detached vitreous cortex from the retinal surface leaving an optically empty subhyaloid space, enhancing its visibility. Ocular movements are also helpful in analyzing intravitreous details. With a swift vitreous movement and a slow return to the original position, the distribution and interrelations of intravitreous opacities are made more visible. Dynamic inspection of the vitreous is therefore necessary to detect these subtle vitreous changes.

9.5 Surgical Treatment for Vitreous Floaters: Important Studies

In 2000 Schiff et al. published an article concerning vitrectomy for persistent vitreous opacities [28]. This article has started a discussion about surgical treatment of mouches volantes, a topic, which was neglected in the past. In this publication, vitrectomy was performed on six patients for persistent visually disturbing vitreous floaters. All patients expressed their satisfaction with the overall postoperative visual function. A quality of life questionnaire indicated that general vision, near vision activities, distance vision activities, mental health and peripheral vision all significantly improved following surgical intervention. Most importantly, no complications occurred.

Since cataract and floaters sometimes coexist in elderly patients, Mossa et al. suggested combined phacoemulsification and deep anterior vitrectomy via a posterior capsulorhexis [20]. They reported on a series of 10 eyes and called this procedure floaterectomy. However, this procedure is not appropriate for the safe and controlled removal of posterior located floaters which are more likely to cause symptoms. Possible intraoperative posterior segment complications cannot be treated adequately with this approach [27].

Roth et al. published a retrospective analysis of 30 phakic (n=17) or pseudophakic (n=13) eyes in which pars plana vitrectomy was performed for persistent vitreous floaters using a 2-port approach and indirect ophthalmoscopy [26]. Patient satisfaction was assessed retrospectively by a self-designed questionnaire. In one pseudophakic patient a retinal detachment occured 48 months postoperatively, otherwise no severe complications were observed during a median follow up period of 20 months. All patients were satisfied with their overall visual function. The authors concluded that vitrectomy is a safe and effective primary treatment for visually disturbing floaters. Similarly, Delaney et al. described one retinal detachment in a series of 15 eyes undergoing vitrectomy for vitreous floaters [5]. Quintyn and Brasseur reported on 4 patients with vitreous floaters and observed no complications after vitrectomy [25].

9.6 Vitrectomy for Vitreous Floaters Despite Full Visual Acuity

Just like many other surgeons [5, 12, 25, 26, 28], we have operated on several patients with vitreous floaters after convincing argumentation of the severity of their symptoms [11]. The unique characteristic in the presented case series is that all patients usually had a full visual acuity (20/20).

9.6.1 Patients

Nine eyes of 8 patients with full visual acuity and minimal objectively detectable pathology underwent vitrectomy for visually disturbing vitreous opacities. In contrast to Schiff's study, only patients with full visual acuity and also phakic eyes were included. Furthermore, not all floaters were clearly visible on ophthalmoscopy. All eyes had a corrected visual acuity of 20/20 or better. Patients were examined on multiple visits to be certain that the symptoms were not improving and to provide detailed information to each patient of the potential risks of the planned vitrectomy. The median duration of symptoms was 12 months. The age of our patients ranged from 40 to 71 years (median age of 57 years). Patients underwent a complete ophthalmic examination. The vitreous and retina were carefully examined by slitlamp biomicroscopy and indirect ophthalmoscopy.

In 6 of the 9 eyes the posterior vitreous was detached on fundus biomicroscopy and ultrasound B examination. Typically the vitreous opacities were minimal, barely visible on photographic documentation (Fig. 9.1) and in marked contrast to patient complaints. The patients in our series were unusually highly differentiated having a high demand on their vision. Their professions included a molecular biologist, a truckdriver, a professor and a technical graphic designer. Symptoms reported by the patients in this series included intermittent blurring, glare or mobile opacities of changing intensity increasing in front of bright backgrounds, visual irritations and difficulties in their daily activities. Despite the high level of visual acuity patients complained about their inability to read continously. When opacities entered the visual axis, they needed to blink, to move their eye or to turn their head to move the opacity out of view. A few of them reported that sudden obscuration or glare lead to delayed reactions in critical situations such as traffic, making it difficult to maintain a customary level of functioning. Given the mild degree of opacification and the patient's overwhelming complaints, the decision for vitrectomy was sometimes hard to make.

9.6.2 Surgical Technique

The surgical technique, a standard pars plana vitrectomy, is not controversial except for one issue; whether the creation of a posterior vitreous detachment is neccessary or not in this group of

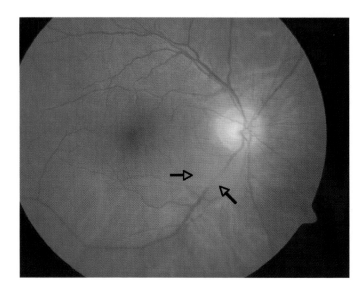

Fig. 9.1 Posterior located symptomatic vitreous opacity (*arrow*) in the central visual field

patients. PVD is associated with the increased risk of iatrogenic retinal tears and, if undetected, a higher rate of postoperative retinal detachment. In most of our patients (6 of the 9 eyes) the posterior hyaloid was already detached preoperatively. In patients with attached posterior hyaloid no PVD was intentionally induced and only a core vitrectomy was performed. In 2 pseudophakic eyes a posterior capsulotomy was made using the vitreous cutter.

9.6.3 Results

The surgical procedure was technically uncomplicated in all patients. No severe postoperative complications occured in our small group of patients. Nuclear sclerosis requiring lens removal developed in 2 of 5 phakic patients. These two patients were 50 and 57 years old. In 3 younger phakic patients (40 years, 40 years, 46 years) no cataract progression was observed during the follow up period of 13 months and VA remained stable. No cataract surgery related complications occured.

All patients expressed their subjective satisfaction and a marked improvement within a few weeks following surgery. Glare was reduced, visual obscuration and irritations abated and they reported a marked improvement in the quality of their professional and private lives.

Objectively, their visual acuity – tested with standardized methods – had remained the same. Two patients who underwent cataract extraction, stated that this complication and the subsequent operation would not have changed their initial decision for the vitrectomy. No PVD occured in the follow-up period in any of the 3 eyes having an attached posterior hyaloid prior to surgery.

9.6.4 Case Report

The following case is representative for the patients that underwent vitrectomy for symptomatic vitreous floaters.

A 57-year-old male professor of agriculture presented with a 9-months history of visually disturbing floaters in his emmetropic right eye. He reported diminished productivity and inability to read for extended periods. Ocular history was otherwise unremarkable. On initial ophthalmic examination, best corrected visual acuity was 20/20 in both eyes. No sign of uveitis was present in the anterior and posterior vitreous. Biomicroscopy revealed no PVD. A few lacunae and fibrous opacities were detected after ocular movements. Indirect ophthalmoscopy revealed no peripheral retinal breaks or degenerations. A core vitrectomy was performed. The patient`s symptoms disappeared within days after surgery. Seven months later uncomplicated cataract extraction was performed and VA was 20/20. The vitreous cavity was clear and no subsequent PVD has developed. The postoperative course was unremarkable and 9 months following the vitrectomy the patient reports absence of preoperative symptoms and markedly improved functioning in all tasks.

9.7 Analysis of Clinical Studies

What is the central question that we can answer after the analysis of previously published small case series and our small group of patients? Due to the small number of patients included we most certainly can not comment on the frequency rate of complications. A much higher complication rate after pars plana vitrectomy for secondary vitreous opacities due to branch retinal vein occlusion, uveitis, vasculitis, sickle cell retinopathy and other severe ocular disorders was reported in an early article of Peyman et al. published in 1976 [23]. In these early vitrectomy years complications of vitrectomy were markedly higher than nowadays with markedly improved instrumentation and techniques. But this experience caused the very restraining and conservative indication for vitrectomy in eyes with good visual acuity. Today, iatrogenic tears, retinal detachment and other complications in this group of patients seem to be low, but will definitely occur with increasing number of patients.

The central question in the opinion of the author is, whether we should offer vitrectomy to patients with subjectively marked visual disturbances despite full visual acuity and minimal objective findings. Is it justified to reject vitrectomy and the reported subjective visual improvement at this low complication rate or do we support a trend of irresponsible life style surgery?

The opinions of various vitreoretinal surgeons regarding this issue will probably markedly differ and without a larger trial including quality-of-life tests we will not be able to answer this question. In this situation guidelines could help in the decision-making process. They should include ocular parameters to minimize the risk of intra- or postoperative complications and also other factors to avoid aggravation of symptoms or hypochondria. Furthermore such guidelines should allow for the fact that symptoms caused by mouches volantes may improve spontaneously over time.

9.8 Alternative Therapeutic Options

Neodym-YAG laser has been used to disrupt localized vitreous opacities in symptomatic patients, but may require multiple sessions [1, 6, 8, 13, 31]. Some patients report the continued presence of smaller annoying opacities despite laser treatment. The procedure is less effective when opacities are not localized, but rather diffuse and a greater application of energy is necessary in the presence of lenticular opacities. Potential complications include retinal and choroidal haemorrhages and damage to the retinal pigment epithelium [1, 6, 13, 24]. Therefore, opacities in the posterior vitreous and lying close to the retina which are most likely to cause symptoms, should not be treated by this method.

Delaney et al. compared Nd:YAG vitreolysis (n=39) and pars plana vitrectomy (n=15) for the treatment of vitreous floaters [5]. Only one third of patients treated with the laser judged the procedure as moderately effective while the majority found no improvement. Vitrectomy, however, achieved superior results.

Summary for the Clinician

- No vitrectomy in patients with acute PVD or a short history of symptoms.
- Repeated follow up visits, at least two, within several months to better estimate the psychological strain traits of the affected and to see if symptoms abate with time.
- Thorough explanation by the surgeon about possible intra- and postoperative complications and subsequent mandatory signed informed consent from the patient.
- Iatrogenic cataract induction and risk factors of cataract extraction have to be discussed together with the possible arising refractive problems especially in younger patients.
- A longer time-interval should be chosen between the preoperative visit of the patient, informed consent and the surgical intervention.
- Preoperative assessment of patients with floaters should include a thorough examination of the vitreous in search of a PVD. Reduced funduscopic view due to cataract or opacities may require complementary ultrasound B-scan examination.
- A careful pre- and intraoperative fundus examination of the peripheral retina is mandatory.
- Patients with ocular risk factors such as untreated retinal holes and equatorial degenerations or with a history of retinal detachment in the second eye should be excluded.
- Detached posterior hyaloid on B-scan ultrasound and pseudophakia are pro arguments in support of surgical intervention.
- Attached posterior hyaloid and phakia are arguments against surgical intervention.
- Intraoperative creation of a posterior vitreous detachment should be avoided.

9.9 Personality Traits

Vitreoretinal surgeons are not as familiar with the treatment of patients having full visual acuity in absence of vision threatening ocular disease as refractive surgeons who are used to dealing with patients having high visual expectations. In most reports on vitrectomy treatment for floaters the high proportion of sophisticated patients was emphasized [11, 26, 28]. Roth et al. reported an appoximate doubling of the proportion of academics in comparison to the population as a whole [26]. This may indicate that the subjective psychological strain is partly related to the educational level and a high requirement on vision.

Some personality traits may be a factor in the perception of visual disturbance caused by vitreous opacities and the desire to have them treated by vitrectomy. Patients tend to be intelligent, observant, and exacting in their description of symptomatology. Specific personality profiles seem to be more prone to disturbances by floaters. Vitrectomy can be very effective in these patients and achieve a complete return to their highly productive lifestyles.

However, the ophthalmologist is not well trained in distinguishing different personality profiles or possible psychiatric disorders. Also patients with somatic disorders may concentrate on vitreous floaters and aggravate their symptoms. These patients would certainly not profit from vitrectomy. A specialist in this field could help to exclude these patients, but many ophthalmologists would not like to convince their patients of the necessity to see a psychiatrist. Therefore, to avoid misestimation, a broad experience, an understanding of human nature of the human condition together with skilled instinct are prerequisites of vitreo retinal surgeons in order to ensure appropiate surgical intervention.

9.10 Alternative Assessment of Visual Function

Snellen visual acuity is the most widely used measure of vision testing. This parameter is often misleading in patients with visually disturbing vitreous floaters. Floaters are not recognized as a disease. The clinician cannot understand the complaints of affected patients who then feel frustrated and misunderstood. Other measures, including contrast sensitivity, stereopsis, reading speed, colour discrimination, visual field, and glare testing, have demonstrated that visual acuity is a descriptor of one simple aspect of vision rather than a comprehensive assessment of visual function.

Standard clinical tests, such as Snellen visual acuity, are unable to quantify many aspects of a visual disturbance and how the disability interferes with day-to-day functioning and overall quality of life. Nevertheless, objective testing is necessary to help quantify the degree of disability and to define criteria used to recommend surgical intervention. Further tests should be established that may allow objective quantification of visual disturbances by various floaters. An approach that is gaining popularity is the use of standardized vision-related quality-of-life instruments to measure the functional visual status of patients [10]. Together with other vision descriptors these tests may be better able to monitor and assess how vitrectomy affects overall visual function, the level of patient satisfaction and lifestyle. Several such instruments have been developed [3, 17, 18, 30]. Two of these tools, the National Eye Institute Visual Function Questionnaire (NEIVFQ-39) and the Visual Function Index (VF-14) have gained increasing acceptance. The NEIVFQ was designed as a comprehensive functional assessment, applicable to various sight-limiting diseases. The VF-14 is an index of visual function that was designed to assess patients undergoing cataract surgery [30]. The format has made it popular because of its high rate of patient compliance. Its validity has also been shown in patients with retinal diseases [17].

To assess the functional outcome in patients with vitreous opacities and patient satisfaction following vitrectomy Schiff et al. performed three quality of life tests. They indicated that general vision, near vision activities, distance vision activities, mental health and peripheral vision all significantly improved following surgical intervention [28].

Table 9.1 Demographic data, pre- and postoperative findings and follow up of vitrectomized patients for vitreous opacities despite full visual acuity. *RE* right eye, *LE* left eye, *ph* phakic, *ps* pseudophakic, *VA* visual acuity, *vy* vitrectomy

Patient Age Gender Eye	Status of the lens	Duration of symptoms (months)	Status of the vitreous posterior hyaloid	Previous ocular history	Refraction	VA pre- Vy	VA post- Vy	Follow-Up period and complications
BJ 57, man, RE	ph	9	Attached	–	Emmetrope	0.9	1.0	9 months / phaco
KM 40, man, LE	ph	12	Attached	–	Emmetrope	1.0	1.0	10 months
KM 40, man, RE	ph	18	Attached	–	Emmetrope	1.0	1.0	13 months
BM 50, man, RE	ph	6	Detached	Cat extraction	Emmetrope	1.0	1.0	15 months / phaco
KH 51, man, RE	ps	6	Detached	Cat extraction	Axial myopia (24.10mm) prior to phaco	1.0	1.0	17 months
NHW 65, man, RE	ps	29	Detached	Cat extraction, YAG capsulotomy	Emmetrope prior to phaco	1.0	1.0	6 months
PD 71, woman, RE	ps	12	Detached	Cat extraction	Emmetrope prior to phaco	1.0pp	0.9	6 months
MK 46, woman, LE	ph	6	Detached	–	Emmetrope	1.0	1.0	15 months
KM 62, man, LE	ps	6	Detached	Cat extraction	Emmetrope (23.17 mm), prior to phaco	1.0	1.0	14 months

9

9.11 Conclusions

Since the start of vitreoretinal surgery not only have vitrectomy techniques and instruments improved but, with the developments in the medical field, the expectations and demands of individuals on quality of life have also increased. In an era in which an increasing number of patients elect surgical interventions such as plastic or refractive surgery, the question is justified as to whether an indication for vitrectomy of vitreous floaters can be established or not.

Few patients with vitreous floaters ultimately require vitrectomy despite good visual acuity. Pars plana vitrectomy seems to be a safe and viable intervention in affected patients. Surgical intervention can result in substantial subjective improvement and increased productivity. With careful case selection, these benefits may outweigh the risks of the procedure. At a time when health care costs comprise a large part of the gross domestic product in industrial countries, it is critical to know what is of value to patients and what is not. Good vision confers a substantially higher quality of life from the patient preference based perspective. Individuals with ocular disease and good visual function have a higher time trade off utility value, and thus a better associated quality of life. This is an important factor to keep in mind when assessing the value and cost effectiveness of vitrectomy. The indication of vitrectomy for floaters opens discussion about a new paradigm of thought concerning the nature and value of health care in vitreoretinal surgery in patients with symptomatic and disturbing floaters. Affected patients are often very productive individuals and seem to profit from vitrectomy. Surgical intervention may add highly leveraged not economic value to individuals`lives, hence to society, and consequently surgical intervention has human and economic value. Therefore, quality of life instruments have to receive more attention in evaluating visual function and should be an essential part of future studies concerning vitrectomy for vitreous floaters.

References

1. Aron-Rosa D, Greenspan DA (1985) Neodymium:YAG laser vitreolysis. Int Ophthalmol Clin 25:125–134

2. Berman ER, Michaelson IC (1964) The chemical composition of the human vitreous body as related to age and myopia. Exp Eye Res 3:9–15

3. Brown MM, Brown GC, Sharma S, et al. (2001) Quality-of-life associated with unilateral and bilateral good vision. Ophthalmology 108:643–647

4. Chignell A (1996) Floaters after cataract surgery. J R Soc Med 89 (6):332

5. Delaney YM, Oyinloye A, Benjamin L (2002) Nd:YAG vitreolysis and pars plana vitrectomy: surgical treatment for vitreous floaters. Eye 16 (1):21–26

6. Fankhauser F, Kwasniewski SF, van der Zypen E (1985) Vitreolysis with the Q-switched laser. Arch Ophthalmol 103:1166–1171

7. Foos RY, Roth AM (1973) Surface structure of the optic nerve head. II. Vitreopapillary attachments and posterior vitreous detachment. Am J Ophthalmol 76:662–671

8. Gandhi JS (2003) Nd:YAG vitreolysis as a treatment for vitreous floaters. Eye 17(1):113

9. Grossniklaus HE, Green WR (1992) Pathological findings in pathologic myopia. Retina 12:127–133

10. Hirneiß C, Neubauer AS, Welge-Lüßen U, et al. (2003) Bestimmung der Lebensqualität des Patienten in der Augenheilkunde. Ophthalmologe 100:1091–1097

11. Hoerauf H, Müller M, Laqua H (2003) Mouches volantes und Vitrektomie bei vollem Visus? Ophthalmologe 100:639–643

12. Hong PH, Han DP, Burke JM, Wirostho WJ (2001) Vitrectomy for large vitreous opacity in retinitis pigmentosa. Am J Ophthalmol 131:133–134

13. Jampol LM, Goldberg MF, Jednock N (1983) Retinal damage from a Q-switch YAG laser. Am J Ophthalmol 96:326–329

14. Kanski JJ (1975) Complications of acute posterior vitreous detachment. Am J Ophthalmol 80:44–46

15. Laqua H (1993) Pars plana-Vitrektomie. In: Wollensak J (ed) Ophthalmochirurgische Komplikationen. Enke, Stuttgart, pp 201–216

16. Linder B (1966) Acute posterior vitreous detachment and its retinal complications. Acta Ophthalmol Suppl 87

17. Linder M, Chang TS, Scott IU, et al. (1999) Validity of the Visual Function Index (VF-14) in patients with retinal disease. Arch Ophthalmol 117:1611–1616

18. Mangione CM, Berry S, Spritzer K, et al (1998) Identifying the content area for the 51st National Eye Institute Visual Function Questionnaire. Arch Ophthalmol 116:227–233

19. Morita H, Funata M, Tokoro T (1995) A clinical study of the development of posterior vitrous detachment in high myopia. Retina 15(2):117–124

20. Mossa F, Delaney YM, Rosen PH, et al. (2002) Floaterectomy: combined phacoemulsification and deep anterior vitrectomy. J Cataract Refract Surg 28(4):589–592

21. Murakami K, Jalkh AE, Avila MP, et al. (1983) Vitreous floaters. Ophthalmology 90:1271–1276

22. Noda S, Hayasaka S, Setogawa T (1993) Patients with asteroid hyalosis and visible floaters. Jpn J Ophthalmol 37:452–455

23. Peyman GA, Huamonte FU, Goldberg MF (1976) Pars plana vitrectomy. Vitrectomy treatment of vitreous opacities. Trans Am Acad Ophthalmol Otolaryngol 81(3Pt1):394–398

24. Puliafito CA, Wasson PJ, Steinert RF (1984) Neodymium-YAG laser surgery on experimental vitreous membrane. Arch Ophthalmol 102:843–847

25. Quintyn JC, Brasseur G (2004) Place de la vitrectomie dans le traitement des corps flottants intravitreens. J Fr Ophtalmol 27(5):491–495

26. Roth M, Trittibach P, Koerner F, Sarra G (2005) Pars-plana-Vitrektomie bei idiopathischen Glaskörpertrübungen. Klin Monatsbl Augenheilkd 222:728–732

27. Sandhya V, Shafquat S (2003) Floaterectomy. J Cataract Refract Surg 29(8):1466–1467

28. Schiff WM, Chang S, Mandava N, Barile GR (2000) Pars plana vitrectomy for persistent, visually significant vitreous opacities. Retina 20:591–596

29. Sebag J (1989) The Vitreous (structure, function, pathobiology). New York Berlin Heidelberg: Springer, pp 73–95

30. Steinberg EP, Tielsch JM, Schein OD et al. (1994) The VF-14: an index of functional impairment in cataract patients. Arch Ophthalmol 112:630–638

31. Tsai WF, Chen YC, Su CY (1993) Treatment of vitreous floaters with neodymium:YAG laser. Br J Ophthalmol 77:485–488

9

Chapter 10

Treatment of Retinal Detachment from Inferior Breaks with Pars Plana Vitrectomy

10

Vicente Martinez-Castillo, Jose Garcia-Arumi,
Anna Boixadera, Miguel A. Zapata

Core Messages

- Vitrectomy is increasingly used as the first approach in patients with rhegmatogenous retinal detachment.
- When primary vitrectomy is used for retinal detachment arising from retinal breaks from the inferior retina, traditionally scleral buckling was also applied to support these breaks; the concern has been that gas tamponade would not support breaks situated in the inferior fundus.
- Recent literature has shown that scleral buckling might not be necessary. Other papers have demonstrated that head-down posturing is also not required.

- Laser can create a watertight seal around retinal breaks during the first postoperative hours.
- Vitrectomy and air alone can be effective in the management of phakic and pseudophakic retinal detachment.
- The following cases should be excluded: Asymptomatic inferior detachments, retinoschisis, pediatric inferior retinal detachments, retinal dialysis, giant tears and proliferative vitreoretinopathy.
- Drainage of subretinal fluid is important and is facilitated by perfluorocarbon liquids.
- Trans-scleral diodes and endolasers (diode and argon) are used and care is taken to surround the edge of all the breaks.

10.1 Introduction

10.1.1 Basics

Inferior breaks are retinal breaks located between 4 and 8 o'clock. They can be classified according to their size, shape (horseshoe tears or atrophic holes), number, and position relative to the equator (anterior or posterior to the equator and equatorial breaks).

Inferior retinal breaks can originate different types of rhegmatogenous retinal detachments (RRDs). RRD can be clinical or subclinical depending on the presence of a posterior vitreous detachment or vitreous syneresis, and on the size of the retinal break. In addition, inferior breaks can be found in combination with superior retinal breaks.

In this chapter the concept of inferior breaks refers only to retinal breaks occurring in primary RRD (Fig. 10.1). Retinal detachment with signs of

10

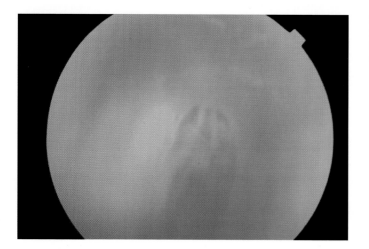

Fig. 10.1 Preoperative illustration of a horseshoe tear located anterior to the equator at 7 o'clock

grade B or greater proliferative vitreoretinopathy [13], giant tears, chronic inferior retinal detachment, and redetachment will not be discussed in this chapter.

10.1.2 Importance of Inferior Breaks When Pars Plana Vitrectomy is Performed

Pars plana vitrectomy (PPV) is increasingly used for primary repair of pseudophakic retinal detachment [1–22]. The development of wide-angle viewing systems and improvements in vitrectomy instrumentation have contributed to expanding the role of PPV in the management of RRD. At the end of the surgical procedure the vitreous cavity is filled with a tamponade agent (air, gas or silicone oil) to allow sufficient time for chorioretinal adhesion to develop and avoid seepage of fluid through the causative break [5, 20].

Postoperative morbidity increases when there are breaks located in an inferior position. Traditionally, inferior breaks present a surgical challenge because it is believed that intraocular gas tamponade cannot provide direct support to the inferior retina. In order to achieve an effective tamponade for retinal breaks, mandatory face-down positioning for 10 days is recommended [20]. To solve this problem, various authors have combined PPV with scleral buckling [1, 3, 7, 8]. On the basis of results from a recent pilot study,

we reported that lengthy face-down positioning is not necessary in pseudophakic retinal detachment [15]. To better understand this approach, we should first review the development of a chorioretinal scar around the retinal break.

10.1.3 Development of a Chorioretinal Scar

A critical step in retinal detachment repair is the development of the chorioretinal scar around the retinal break. The most important effect of chorioretinal adhesion in closing the retinal break is to induce a watertight seal that prevents seepage of vitreous fluid into the subretinal space [5, 23]. Although the mechanism producing the laser-induced bond within the first days after photocoagulation is uncertain, histologic studies have shown that a proteinaceous coagulum develops at the interface between the retina and the retinal pigment epithelium, followed by cicatricial adhesion due to proliferation and migration of glial cells into the wound site [6, 12, 24].

In clinical practice, a correlation with these histologic findings can be established postoperatively. During the first 5 days, the laser spots are surrounded by retinal edema (Fig.10.2a). Over the following 7 days, the retinal edema disappears (Fig. 10.2b). Finally, in the second week, a chorioretinal scar develops (Fig. 10.2c). During this period the strength of the chorioretinal adhesion increases. However, experimental studies have shown that fresh laser burns produce a greater than normal adhesive bond between the retina and retinal pigment epithelium 24 h post-treatment. Hence, the role of the surgical technique lies in the development of a sealed chorioretinal adhesion during the first hours postoperatively to obviate the need for face-down positioning. Once the chorioretinal adhesion is sealed, a chorioretinal scar will develop postoperatively.

10.1.4 Type of Tamponade Agent for Inferior Breaks

The ability of tamponade agents to avoid seepage of fluid through the retinal breaks depends on the interaction of three factors: the aqueous phase, the tamponade agent and the retina [5, 23]. The rationale for using a long-term tamponade for managing inferior breaks in PPV is based on the theory that the intraocular gas bubble will prevent intravitreal fluid from entering the break and accumulating in the subretinal space. However, as was mentioned above, the critical step is the development of a sealed chorioretinal adhesion

during the first postoperative hours. The need for short- or long-term postoperative tamponading depends on two factors related to the pars plana vitrectomy technique: the use of perfluoro-N-octane and the care with which vitreous dissection is performed around the retinal breaks. The better the peripheral vitreous dissection around the breaks, the shorter the time that is needed to create a sealed chorioretinal adhesion.

10.2 Management of Inferior Breaks with PPV: Recent Publications

During the last 5 years there has been a change in the surgical management of retinal detachment with inferior breaks by PPV (Table 10.1). This section centers on two schools of thought in this respect. The first advocates the use of scleral buckling combined with PPV. Initially, a case series reported promising results with PPV alone [19] and the initial reattachment rate was 89%. However, this pilot study included only 9 cases, 4 pseudophakic and 5 phakic. Moreover,

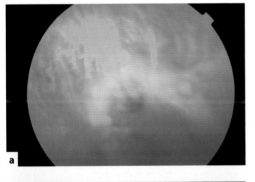

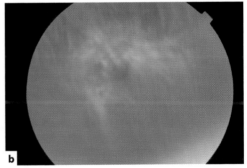

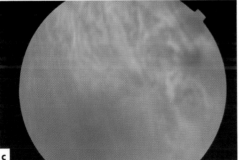

Fig. 10.2 a Second postoperative day. Confluent diode laser spots around the borders of the retinal break and retinal edema are evident. The retina is completely attached. **b** Tenth postoperative day. Retinal edema decreases. Note the change in color of the laser spots. **c** One month postoperatively. A chorioretinal scar has developed around the borders of the retinal break

10

Table 10.1 Rhegmatogenous retinal detachments with inferior breaks managed with pars plana vitrectomy alone

Reference	Year	Number	Inferior breaks	Primary success (%)	Final success (%)	PVR (%)	VA (%)	Tamponade	Postoperative positioning	Study design
[4]	1985	29	2	79	93	7	81 ≥20/50	Air	Yes	Retrospective
[21]	1987	60	3	86	92	0	76≥20/50	SF_6	Yes	Retrospective
[10]	1995	32	Not available	78	94	19	41 ≥20/50	SF_6	Yes	Retrospective
[9]	1996	53	6	64	92	6	41 ≥20/50	SF_6	Yes	Retrospective
[2]	1999	275	Not available	88	96	6	61 ≥20/40	Air, C_3F_8, SF_6	Yes	Prospective
[17]	2000	78	29	94	96	5	Not available	SF_6, C_3F_8,	Yes	Retrospective
[19]	2001	9	9	89	100	0	66.6 ≥20/40	SF_6, C_3F_8, SO	Yes	Prospective
[16]	2004	48	48	81.3	95.8	NA	Not available	SF_6, C_3F_8, SO	Yes	Prospective
[22]	2004	41	41	89	95	5	Not available	SF_6, C_3F_8	Yes	Retrospective
[11]	2004	27	5	89	100		96 ≥20/50	Air	Yes	Prospective
[18]	2004	45	Not available	97.78	100	2.2	Not available	SF_6	Yes	Prospective
[15]	2005	15	15	93.3	100	0	Mean: 20/30	Air	No	Prospective
[14]	2005	40	40	90	100	2.5	Mean: 20/33	Air	No	Prospective

three types of tamponade agents were used, SF_6, C_3F_8, and silicone oil. All the patients underwent postoperative positioning for 10 days. Two recent clinical studies [16, 22] comparing PPV alone versus PPV combined with scleral buckling have shown that anatomic and functional results do not differ between the two groups. Phakic and pseudophakic patients without clinical proliferative vitreoretinopathy were included in these studies, gas tamponade (SF_6 or C_3F_8) was used, and patients were positioned postoperatively.

The second approach refers to the management of inferior breaks with PPV alone and no postoperative positioning [14, 15]. It is important to highlight that only pseudophakic patients without signs of proliferative vitreoretinopathy were included in these studies in order to achieve complete vitreous dissection around the causative retinal breaks located inferiorly. These pilot studies have provided evidence that face-down posture after PPV is not necessary to achieve retinal reattachment in pseudophakic RRD with inferior breaks. Although this issue was not specifically addressed, other authors have reported favorable results with pars plana vitrectomy alone for the management of pseudophakic and aphakic retinal detachment including superior and inferior breaks [2, 18].

10.3 PPV Alone with Air Tamponade: Surgical Technique

10.3.1 Inclusion Criteria

As previously discussed, patients with primary pseudophakic and aphakic retinal detachment are the best candidates for this surgical technique. Asymptomatic inferior RRDs, retinoschisis, pediatric inferior retinal detachments, retinal dialysis, giant tears, and retinal detachments with proliferative vitreoretinopathy should be excluded. The intraoperative number of retinal breaks is an important factor to consider when air is used as a tamponade agent.

10.3.2 Vitrectomy

It is essential to determine the extension of the retinal detachment as well as the number, type, position and size of retinal breaks preoperatively. This information will help us to choose the position of the dominant sclerotomy to accommodate a lighted infusion or a 25-gauge sutureless xenon chandelier light. The main advantage of using these systems for the surgeon is to perform scleral depression with the second hand. In order to maximize vitreous dissection around the retinal breaks the vitreous probe should be opposite to the break.

The first step in this surgical procedure is to perform a careful vitrectomy around the sclerotomy sites to avoid vitreous traction and incarceration during the surgical procedure. Then, it is essential to perform meticulous vitreous dissection. The sclerotomy site must be located opposite the causative break(s).

Summary for the Clinician

- Peripheral vitreous dissection around the causative breaks is essential when using an air tamponade agent without postoperative prone positioning.
- Vitreous dissection should be performed under scleral depression.

10.3.3 Drainage of Subretinal Fluid

The subretinal fluid is drained with the use of perfluorocarbon (PFCL) liquids. There are two main reasons why this agent is applied: to secure the equatorial and peripheral retina, thereby allowing further vitreous dissection and reducing the risk of enlarging the break (in addition, the retinal breaks are marked with diode laser spots under PFCL) and to create an apposition between the border of the retinal breaks and the retinal pigment epithelium before fluid/air exchange (Fig. 10.3a). To maximize subretinal fluid drainage, fluid–air exchange is performed with a silicone tip through the most posterior causative break (Fig. 10.3b).

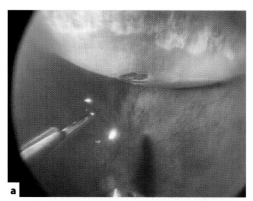

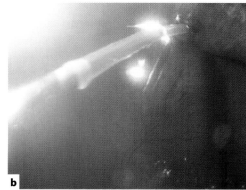

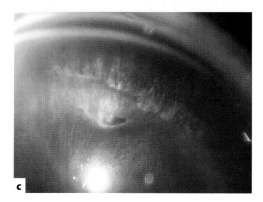

Fig. 10.3 a Surgeon's view. The meniscus of the perfluorocarbon liquid reaches the posterior border of the causative break. Peripheral vitreous dissection is performed under scleral depression. **b** Fluid–air exchange is performed with a silicone-tipped cannula. Subretinal fluid is drained through the causative break. **c** Surgeon's view. Trans-scleral diode laser photocoagulation is performed

10.3.4 Retinopexy

The success of the surgical procedure depends on correct photocoagulation of all the retinal breaks. Laser marks are very useful to precisely identify the retinal breaks. Identification under air is more complex, particularly when the causative retinal breaks are small. The main aspects to be considered are the following:

- The borders of the retinal breaks must be precisely identified.
- Retinopexy is performed with a trans-scleral or endo-laser (Fig. 10.3C). Two types of lasers are currently used, a diode laser or an argon laser. The laser spots are confluent and the energy is increased by intervals of 50 mW if no tissue effect is observed.
- Retinopexy is always performed after fluid/air exchange to avoid contact of subretinal fluid with the treated retinal borders.

Summary for the Clinician

- The use of perfluorocarbon liquids allows dissection of the anterior vitreous and vitreous around the retinal break.
- Retinopexy must be performed carefully around the borders of the retinal break(s).
- Identification of retinal breaks is more difficult in cases with a broken posterior capsule or posterior capsule opacification. In these cases, retinopexy can be performed under perfluorocarbon liquid.

10.3.5 Tamponade Agent

The choice of a tamponade agent (air or gas) does not influence development of a chorioretinal scar around the retinal break with the surgical technique described above. However, if the main steps of the surgical technique cannot be performed properly, then a long-term tamponade agent must be used. The main variables to consider are the surgeon's experience, intraoperative variables, and the characteristics of the retinal detachment. The surgeon's experience is critical to avoid vitreous incarceration, to precisely identify all the retinal breaks, and to perform vitreous dissection. Intraoperative variables include crystalline status, intraoperative mydriasis, posterior capsule opacification, and complete peripheral retinal examination under scleral depression. Retinal detachment characteristics: number, type and size of retinal breaks, presence of proliferative vitreoretinopathy.

The main indication for using a long-term tamponade is primary detachment with difficult intraoperative visualization or complications during the surgical procedure. In these cases the use of a long-term tamponade will allow development of a chorioretinal scar before the tamponade has been absorbed.

Summary for the Clinician

■ The best cases are pseudophakic retinal detachments. In order to use short-term tamponade agents in phakic cases with inferior breaks, meticulous vitreous dissection must be performed around the causative breaks.

References

1. Bartz-Schmidt KU, Kirchhof B, Heimann K. Primary vitrectomy for pseudophakic retinal detachment. Br J Ophthalmol 1996;80:346–349.
2. Campo RV, Sipperley JO, Sneed SR, et al. Pars plana vitrectomy without scleral buckle for pseudophakic retinal detachments. Ophthalmology 1999;106:1811–1815; discussion 1816.
3. Desai UR, Strassman IB. Combined pars plana vitrectomy and scleral buckling for pseudophakic and aphakic retinal detachments in which a break is not seen preoperatively. Ophthalmic Surg Lasers 1997;28:718–722.
4. Escoffery RF, Olk RJ, Grand MG, Boniuk I. Vitrectomy without scleral buckling for primary rhegmatogenous retinal detachment. Am J Ophthalmol 1985;99:275–281.
5. Fawcett IM, Williams RL, Wong D. Contact angles of substances used for internal tamponade in retinal detachment surgery. Graefes Arch Clin Exp Ophthalmol 1994;232:438–444.
6. Folk JC, Sneed SR, Folberg R, et al. Early retinal adhesion from laser photocoagulation. Ophthalmology 1989;96:1523–1525.
7. Gartry DS, Chignell AH, Franks WA, Wong D. Pars plana vitrectomy for the treatment of rhegmatogenous retinal detachment uncomplicated by advanced proliferative vitreoretinopathy. Br J Ophthalmol 1993;77:199–203.
8. Hakin KN, Lavin MJ, Leaver PK. Primary vitrectomy for rhegmatogenous retinal detachment. Graefes Arch Clin Exp Ophthalmol 1993;231:344–346.
9. Heimann H, Bornfeld N, Friedrichs W, et al. Primary vitrectomy without scleral buckling for rhegmatogenous retinal detachment. Graefes Arch Clin Exp Ophthalmol 1996;234:561–568.
10. Höing C, Heidenkummer H-P, Kampik A. Primäre Vitrektomie bei rhegmatogener Ablatio retinae. Ophthalmologe 1995;92:668–671.
11. Hotta K, Sugitani A, Uchino Y. Pars plana vitrectomy without long-acting gas tamponade for primary rhegmatogenous retinal detachment. Ophthalmologica 2004;218:270–273.
12. Kita M, Negi A, Kawano S, Honda Y. Photothermal, cryogenic, and diathermic effects on retinal adhesive force in vivo. Retina 1991;11:441–444.
13. Machemer R, Aaberg TM, Freeman HM, et al. An updated classification of retinal detachment with proliferative vitreoretinopathy. Am J Ophthalmol 1991;112:159–165.
14. Martinez-Castillo V, Boixadera A, Verdugo A, Garcia-Arumi J. Pars plana vitrectomy alone for the management of inferior breaks in pseudophakic retinal detachment without face down position. Ophthalmology 2005;112:1222–1226.
15. Martínez-Castillo V, Verdugo A, Boixadera A, García-Arumí J, Corcóstegui B. Management of inferior breaks in pseudophakic rhegmatogenous retinal detachment with PPV and air. Arch Ophthalmol 2005;123;1078–1081.

16. Sharma A, Grigoropoulos V, Williamson TH. Management of primary rhegmatogenous retinal detachment with inferior breaks. Br J Ophthalmol 2004;88:1372–1375.

17. Speicher M, Fu AD, Martin JP, Von Fricken MA. Primary vitrectomy alone for repair of retinal detachments following cataract surgery. Retina 2000;20:459–464.

18. Stangos A, Petropoulos I, Brozou C, Kapetanios A, Whatham A, Pournaras C. Pars-plana vitrectomy alone vs vitrectomy with scleral buckling for primary rhegmatogenous pseudophakic retinal detachment. Am J Ophthalmol 2004;138:952–958.

19. Tanner V, Minihan M, Williamson TH. Management of inferior retinal breaks during pars plana vitrectomy for retinal detachment. Br J Ophthalmol 2001;85:480–482.

20. Thompson JT. Kinetics of intraocular gases. Disappearance of air, sulfur hexafluoride, and perfluoropropane after pars plana vitrectomy. Arch Ophthalmol 1989;107:687–691.

21. Van Effenterre G, Haut J, Larricart P, et al. Gas tamponade as a single technique in the treatment of retinal detachment: is vitrectomy needed? A comparative study of 120 cases. Graefes Arch Clin Exp Ophthalmol 1987;225:254–258.

22. Wickham L, Connor M, Aylward GW. Vitrectomy and gas for inferior break retinal detachments: are the results comparable to vitrectomy, gas, and scleral buckle? Br J Ophthalmol 2004;88:1376–1379.

23. Williams R, Wong D. The influence of explants on the physical efficiency of tamponade agents. Graefes Arch Clin Exp Ophthalmol 1999;237:870–874.

24. Yoon YH, Marmor MF. Rapid enhancement of retinal adhesion by laser photocoagulation. Ophthalmology 1988;95:1385–1388.

10

Subclinical Retinal Detachment

Jose Garcia-Arumi, Anna Boixadera,
Vicente Martinez-Castillo, Miguel A. Zapata

Core Messages

- Subclinical retinal detachment (SCRD) refers to rhegmatogenous retinal detachment that does not cause changes in the patient's visual field or acuity. The real incidence and natural history of SCRD are unknown because the patients are asymptomatic and do not seek medical care.

- The natural history of SCRD varies between fellow and non-fellow eyes. SCRD progresses in 50% of fellow eyes; thus, these patients are treated. SCRD extends in only 10% of non-fellow eyes; hence, treatment must be individualized in this group of patients. Superior SCRD in young patients who undertake considerable physical activity and those due to horseshoe-shaped tears might need to be treated. If SCRD is not treated, regular examinations are mandatory.

- SCRD can lead to epimacular proliferation or cystoid macular edema. When treatment is indicated, scleral buckling is the first-choice surgical technique.

11.1 Definition

In 1952, Schepens [29] applied the term "subclinical retinal detachment" (SCRD) to eyes in which the diagnosis of rhegmatogenous retinal detachment (RRD) could not be made with the usual methods of investigation. In 1958 [30], this author defined the term differently, as follows: "retinal detachment that is so peripheral and so flat that it does not cause changes in the patient's visual field or acuity." In this second definition the concept was based on the absence of symptoms noted by the patient, in contrast to the first, which depended on the ability of the examiner to discover its presence.

In 1973, Davis [13] restricted the definition by giving it anatomical specificity. It referred to eyes in which the subretinal fluid extended at least one disc diameter (DD) away from the nearest retinal break, but no more than two DDs posterior to the equator. Nonetheless, asymptomatic detachments that extend more posteriorly are sometimes diagnosed as SCRD and managed in the same way [1, 11].

There is no internationally accepted classification system for simple RRDs, although the requirements for describing such detachments in publications have been laid down [36]. Aylward [1] classified retinal detachments according to their extension as limited or extensive, and into three categories according to the type of retinal tear. The term "limited RRD" is used to describe a detachment in which the area of the affected retina does not give rise to significant symptoms, either detected by the patient before the examination or noticed after the physician has informed the patient of the condition. A limited RRD is one that can be left alone without detriment to the patient if there is no chance of progression. In contradistinction to this, an extensive RRD is one in which significant symptoms are detected or can be demonstrated, and which cannot go untreated without leaving the patient with visual morbidity. Some limited detachments are SCRDs.

Aylward's three categories of RRD according to the type of retinal tear include: category 1, RRD secondary to round holes; category 2,

RRD secondary to dialyses; and category 3, RRD secondary to horseshoe-shaped tears [1]. Most SCRD fall into category 1: areas of retinal detachment secondary to an atrophic hole or secondary to small round holes in an area of lattice degeneration. They occur mainly in young myopic patients and are picked up incidentally in a routine examination (Fig. 11.1).

Retinal detachments with a demarcation line are not always SCRDs. It is a misconception that a demarcation line posterior to the area of detachment indicates a safe lesion, since such detachments can progress later on. The demarcation line does mean that the RRD has a duration of at least 3 months and implies stability for at least that period (Fig. 11.2) [33]. In one report the de-

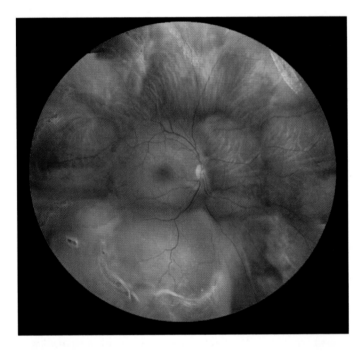

Fig. 11.1 Fundus photograph showing an asymptomatic inferior traumatic rhegmatogenous retinal detachment (RRD) in a 15-year-old myopic woman (-8 diopters) after a contusive trauma. The RRD was secondary to round holes in inferior lattice degeneration. Since it was traumatic in origin and had a high risk of progression, the detachment was treated

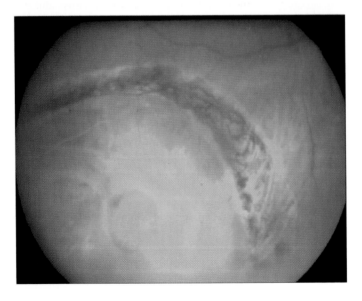

Fig. 11.2 Fundus photograph showing a subclinical retinal detachment (SCRD) secondary to an inferotemporal retinal dialyses in a 20-year-old man. There is a demarcation line at the posterior border of the detachment and secondary retinoschisis. The patient was treated with scleral buckling surgery and cryotherapy

11

marcation line failed to prevent progression in 51 out of 66 cases [3]. In contrast, all the retinal detachments had a demarcation line in a series of SCRD patients [11].

Little attention has been paid to this entity in the literature because most publications combine cases of asymptomatic RRD with symptomatic RRD. The term SCRD does not have the same meaning for all ophthalmologists and this may account for discrepancies regarding the prognosis of this condition and confusion derived from the conclusions of some published reports.

Summary for the Clinician

- Subclinical retinal detachment has been defined as an RRD in which the subretinal fluid extends at least one DD away from the nearest retinal break, but no more than two DD posterior to the equator. In clinical practice subclinical retinal detachment is considered a rhegmatogenous retinal detachment that does not cause changes in the patient's visual field or acuity.
- Most SCRD are secondary to small round holes in young myopic patients, picked up in a routine examination.
- Retinal detachments with a demarcation line are not always SCRD, and the line does not indicate that the lesion will not progress.

11.2 Natural History

It is not possible to know the incidence or the true natural history of SCRD because the patients are asymptomatic and do not seek medical care. The estimates are based on relatively small published series of patients who were diagnosed in a routine ophthalmologic examination.

Much of the understanding of the natural history of RRD, retinal breaks and other lesions comes from the careful work of Norman Byer [7]. In his long-term follow-up of patients with asymptomatic retinal breaks, 17 eyes with 18 areas of SCRD were diagnosed. He also described the natural history of SCRD [7] and found an 11%

risk of progression from subclinical to clinical RRD. This rate of progression is exactly equal to the likelihood of spontaneous regression and disappearance of this type of RRD, found in 11% of patients who received no treatment [9]. Regarding the location of the lesion, most SCRD (59%) were inferior and 90.9% were in the temporal half of the fundus; this location may have contributed to maintaining the RRD subclinically. The rate of progression to clinical RRD was calculated to be less than 1% per year and myopic females were found to have a 4.7 times greater risk of developing SCRD than males. The author concluded that compared with clinical RRD, SCRD is much less threatening to the vision and health of the eye in phakic non-fellow eyes. In the cases in which SCRD progressed, none of the patients lost vision as a result of the initial decision to defer surgery.

Most cases of SCRD develop early in adult life, with 45% occurring in patients under the age of 27. Therefore, if an average of 1% risk of progression per year is applied to a 25-year-old, then the risk of progression of SCRD to clinical RRD over an 80-year total life span would be 55%. Of course, these figures are the result of extrapolating the trends found in Byer's study (with a mean follow-up of 13.5 years) over the lifetime of a patient, which is risky. Unfortunately, there are no studies providing data for SCRD in eyes followed up for 40 or 50 years, and this information is necessary to determine the true cumulative risk of developing clinical RRD over the life of the patient. According to Dr. Byer's data, routine treatment would not be justified, but patients should be re-examined annually or at more frequent intervals if changes are observed. If there is progression to clinical RRD, surgical treatment would be justified. In Byer's paper the cases of SCRD were in non-fellow eyes. An earlier study involving fellow eyes [12] suggested that the risk of SCRD progression is about 50%. Thus, the natural history seems to be completely different in this higher risk group and treatment would be indicated from the time SCRD is diagnosed.

11.2.1 Role of the Vitreous

An important issue that probably affects the natural history of SCRD is the state of the vitreous. It has been observed that most cases of SCRD are secondary to atrophic holes or round holes in lattice degeneration. In most of these cases there is no posterior vitreous detachment [35]. In SCRD, the absence of posterior vitreous detachment is likely to prevent the retinal detachment from extending. Some authors have observed, however, that even when posterior vitreous detachment develops most cases of SCRD do not progress [35].

Summary for the Clinician

- It is not possible to know the true incidence and natural history of SCRD since patients are asymptomatic and do not seek medical care.
- The natural history is different in fellow and non-fellow eyes. In phakic non-fellow eyes, the rate of progression to clinical RRD is less than 1% per year, whereas in fellow eyes it is around 50%.
- It is likely that the absence of posterior vitreous detachment in most cases of SCRD helps to limit progression.

11.3   Therapeutic Options

11.3.1   Observation

The related literature includes helpful data for assessing the risk of treatment versus follow-up for asymptomatic RRD. If the progression rate of SCRD is as low as reported [8], a surgical intervention may not be advisable. Brod et al. [6] followed-up 28 patients (31 eyes) with asymptomatic RRD for mean of 3.4 years (0.5 to 12.1 years) and observed progression of the detachment in only 2 of 31 eyes (6%). The majority occurred in myopic patients, 76% had a refractive error of −2 diopters or more, and 74% showed a demarcation line. Greven et al. [17] evaluated the results of treating asymptomatic RRDs with a scleral buckle and reported retinal reattachment in 28 of 28 eyes (100%) undergoing one procedure. Visual acuity was stable or improved in 93% of eyes.

Indirect laser photocoagulation can be used in smaller SCRDs, whereas larger lesions require a scleral buckle or pneumatic retinopexy, which are more costly and carry a higher associated risk of complications than photocoagulation. Dr. Byer advocates indefinite follow-up in these patients to detect changes in the SCRD [8]. Some authors [31] have disputed this approach on the basis that the cost of annual examinations by a retina specialist would approach the cost of a surgical procedure, considering that the hypothetical 25-year-old patient would be monitored for around 55 additional years of life. If this same patient were treated with laser photocoagulation, a scleral buckle, or pneumatic retinopexy, there would be no need for follow-up by a specialist several years after the diagnosis. An evidence-based analysis might help us to more precisely define the benefits and costs of SCRD follow-up versus treatment.

Cohen [11] described a series of 18 patients with SCRD, but the definition of the condition used in his report does not adhere to Davis' criteria; retinal detachments extending more than 2 DD posterior to the equator are also included. Most cases of SCRD were secondary to retinal holes, 8 out of the 18 patients had myopia, and all had a partial demarcation line at presentation. RRD advanced in only one patient and then remained stable and asymptomatic during the 4 years of follow-up.

Many surgeons recommend routine examinations at regular intervals, for example, every 6 months or annually. However, signs of progression are most likely to occur between follow-up examinations, and if the patient is unable to detect a change, there is a risk that the macula will detach before treatment can be applied, with a potential for worse visual outcome than would be expected if the patient had received surgical treatment initially.

When adopting a conservative approach to cases such as these, it is important to consider other factors in addition to the characteristics of the detachment, including the required periods of observation and the patients' ability to attend urgently if they experience symptoms. The demands of physical activity and the need for intraocular surgery are also important, as are situations involving unusual external forces on the vitreous body, as occurs in space travel, which could lead to symptomatic retinal detachment.

When contemplating treatment, several factors must be taken into consideration, such as the location of the SCRD. When the lesion is in a superior position, treatment should be undertaken since subretinal fluid from superior tears spreads more rapidly than from inferior ones due to the forces of gravity. The type of retinal tear may also be important for the treatment decision. SCRD secondary to horseshoe-shaped tears are exceptional, since most of these are associated with symptomatic posterior vitreous detachment. However, when they occur, they tend to progress rapidly since most of them involve significant traction on the tear flap; hence, observation may not be the optimal approach for this type of SCRD.

The risk of observation must be balanced against the risks of surgical complications, particularly in this category of detachment. If SCRD is left untreated, contact between the retinal pigment epithelium and the vitreous cavity will act as a stimulus for epimacular proliferation or cystoid macular edema, and both can decrease visual acuity. On the other hand, surgery may cause chronic discomfort, diplopia or visual loss. All these factors should be fully discussed with the patient.

Thanks to Dr. Byer's efforts, the physician can inform the patient of the 1% risk per year of progression to clinical RRD and encourage the patient to make the decision. The available data demonstrate that the decision to treat or follow-up SCRD is not urgent and can be made without pressuring toward a surgical intervention unless the patient has had RRD in the fellow eye.

11.3.2 Laser Demarcation

The area of detached retina can be effectively limited by creating a band of chorioretinal adhesion completely surrounding the detachment. There is evidence that adhesion between the retina and the retinal pigment epithelium begins to develop 24 h after treatment [15]. However, it takes 3 to 14 days to achieve maximum strength [41]. Laser demarcation does nothing to resolve an existing detachment and when it is performed, the over-

lying nerve fiber layers in the area of the laser are rendered dysfunctional. Although cryotherapy can be used in these patients, laser photocoagulation is preferred since it causes less tissue damage and inflammatory side effects to the external eye.

11.3.3 Surgery

The anatomical results of surgery are expected to be good, and are similar to those of macula-on retinal detachment, but there is the risk of additional ocular morbidity. Tillery and Lucier [32] reported the results of buckling surgery in patients with detachment secondary to round holes in lattice degeneration (some of whom were asymptomatic). The reattachment rate was 98%; however, 15% had poorer postoperative vision.

Greven et al. [17] reported the results of 28 eyes in 27 patients with SCRD. In 16 eyes SCRD was detected during a routine examination and in 8 it occurred in the fellow of an eye with a previous asymptomatic retinal detachment. All but two eyes were treated with a segmental buckle and the remaining two were encircled. Initial reattachment rate was 100%, but one eye developed another detachment associated with a new retinal break 14 months later. In one eye visual acuity decreased from 20/20 to 20/30.

All the surgical techniques usually applied to treat RRD can be used to manage this type of retinal detachment: pneumatic retinopexy, scleral buckling or pars plana vitrectomy.

11.3.3.1 Pneumatic Retinopexy

Pneumatic retinopexy is indicated for cases of SCRD with a superior break. An expanding gas is injected into the vitreous cavity, followed by application of cryotherapy or laser photocoagulation once the retina has reattached, as described by Hilton and Grizzard [22]. The head of the patient is then positioned so that the gas bubble is in apposition to the break or breaks. The most important complications of this technique are elevated intraocular pressure, subretinal gas or new retinal breaks [38].

A prospective randomized trial found that pneumatic retinopexy has a success rate similar to that of vitrectomy with cryotherapy and gas [36]. A prospective comparative controlled trial and a large multicenter randomized trial compared pneumatic retinopexy with scleral buckling and reported a higher rate of primary reattachment in the scleral buckling group: 82 vs. 73% with no significant differences (p>0.05). There were no differences in the final reattachment rates. Nevertheless, patients with pneumatic retinopexy had less morbidity and better final visual acuity [34]. This high reattachment rate is in phakic eyes; the technique is less effective in aphakic or pseudophakic eyes [26]. Advantages of the technique include the fact that it does not induce refractive changes and the lens changes are smaller than in vitrectomy.

11.3.3.2   Scleral Buckling

The aim of buckling surgery is to create an indentation in the sclera beneath the retinal break to reduce the flow of fluid into the subretinal space, thereby leading to resolution of the detachment. The buckle closes the break, but sealing is not achieved until either cryotherapy or laser retinopexy is performed. Limited SCRD can be treated with segmental buckles or radial elements, but some surgeons prefer an encircling band. Encirclement is associated with a higher risk of motility disturbance and refractive changes and can lead to long-term problems like erosion of the buckle through the sclera or conjunctiva. The main advantage of buckling surgery is that it is an extraocular technique.

11.3.3.3   Pars Plana Vitrectomy

Vitrectomy offers a more successful approach for simple detachments with significant vitreous opacity, aphakia or pseudophakia, or with posterior breaks, which would require a large scleral buckle. Other indications include eyes with a thin sclera, which could make scleral buckling dangerous. Pars plana vitrectomy is not routinely indicated in SCRD unless one of the above-mentioned circumstances is present.

The state of the vitreous can also affect the surgical indication. In cases in which the vitreous is attached, the use of vitrectomy can be technically difficult. Often, the status of the vitreous is secondary to the type of retinal break. In a large series of 140 round-hole detachments requiring treatment, only 8 (7%) eyes had a detached vitreous and the associated clinical findings in these cases suggested that the RRD predated the posterior vitreous detachment [35]. The vitreous can also be attached in cases of retinal dialyses. In contrast, posterior vitreous detachment is found in most RRDs with "U" tears.

11.3.4   Pros and Cons of Treating

11.3.4.1   Pros of Treating

- Patients who have physically demanding jobs will not require restriction of their daily activity.
- If treatment is needed many years later, it is likely that photoreceptor degeneration in the detached area of the retina will limit recovery of the visual field, thus reducing the benefits of treatment at that stage.
- Progression is most likely to occur between follow-up examinations, and if the patient is unable to detect a change, there is a risk that the macula will detach before treatment can be applied. Hence, the final vision might be poorer than would have been expected if the patient had received surgical treatment initially.
- Pigment epithelial cells released into the vitreous cavity while the retinal tear remains untreated may be a source of subsequent epimacular proliferation.
- An area of chronic SCRD can cause cystoid macular edema, which can affect visual acuity in the long term.

11.3.4.2   Cons of Treating

- Risk of diplopia, refractive shift, bleeding, choroidal effusion, and extrusion of the explant in scleral buckling surgery.

- Risk of cataract formation, glaucoma, endophthalmitis, iatrogenic retinal tears, cystoid macular edema, macular pucker, and proliferative vitreoretinopathy in cases of pneumatic retinopexy and vitrectomy.

Summary for the Clinician

- The decision to treat or follow-up SCRD is not urgent and can be made without pressuring toward a surgical intervention unless the patient has had an RRD in the fellow eye.
- If observation is chosen, routine examinations at regular intervals are mandatory.
- When deciding whether or not to treat the patient, consider all the situations that could lead to symptomatic RRD (physical activity demand, intraocular surgery, space travel, superior location of the retinal break, and presence of horseshoe-shaped tears) as well as the patient's ability to attend urgently if symptoms appear.
- If the SCRD is treated, scleral buckling is the first-choice option. Risks of surgery need to be discussed with the patient.

11.4 Current Clinical Practice/Recommendations

On the basis of the above information, the following recommendations can be made:
- Indicate treatment in all fellow eyes with SCRD.
- In non-fellow eyes, treat retinal detachments that are superior, secondary to horseshoe-shaped tears, in patients requiring a high level of physical activity and those unable to attend urgently in the case of visual acuity changes.
- As a first line treatment, scleral buckling is indicated. Possible complications need to be discussed with the patient before surgery.
- If left untreated, observation is mandatory. Take into consideration the risk of epimacular proliferation and cystoid macular edema.

11.5 Subclinical Retinal Detachment Diagnosed with Optical Coherence Tomography After Successful Surgery for Rhegmatogenous Retinal Detachment

The introduction of optical coherence tomography (OCT) technology [14, 21, 23] has led to new findings in studies of retinal abnormalities, particularly macular disorders [20, 21, 24, 27, 28, 37].

Persistent foveal subretinal fluid following successful surgery for RRD observed with OCT, but not with ophthalmoscopy, was first reported in 2002 after scleral buckling surgery [18, 19]. The subfoveal clear space observed with OCT was defined as residual subretinal fluid (Fig. 11.3). Although the resolution of the OCT scanner is very fine (10–15 µm), associated artifacts have been reported [10]; hence, OCT findings should be interpreted carefully. The change in the refractive index at an interface is responsible for most of the OCT signal [10], and changes at the borders give off high signals. Cases with residual subretinal fluid have a highly refractive layer at the outer surface of the neurosensory retina and this layer indicates the presence of a refractive index change. Thus, this change seems to indicate the existence of subretinal fluid.

According to Wolfensberger and Gonvers [40], 13 (81%) out of 16 eyes with macula-off RRD had foveal subretinal fluid detected by OCT 1 month after scleral buckling. In their study, visual recovery in eyes with residual subretinal

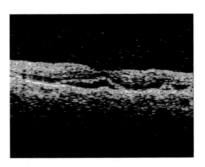

Fig. 11.3 Optical coherence tomography 1 month after successful surgery of a RRD treated with pars plana vitrectomy. Foveal subretinal fluid can be observed

fluid tended to be worse at 1, 6, and 12 months postoperatively than that in eyes with complete foveal retinal reattachment.

In the study of Baba et al. [2], residual foveal subretinal fluid was detected in 9 out of 15 eyes (60%) treated with scleral buckling, a prevalence close to that reported by Wolfensberger [39]. However, according to these authors, residual subretinal fluid did not appear to influence best-corrected visual acuity or improvement of visual acuity 6 months after surgery. In fact, 2 weeks after surgery, visual acuity of eyes with foveal subretinal fluid was unexpectedly better than in those with no subretinal fluid accumulation. In general, visual acuity recovered favorably in all eyes postoperatively.

Wolfensberger et al. [40] reported that persistent subfoveal detachment was only observed after scleral buckling surgery. The authors found that at the first postoperative month, 67% of patients (n=6) treated with scleral buckling showed persistent foveal detachment and 11% (n=1) diffuse detachment. In the pars plana vitrectomy group, all patients (100%) had a flat fovea. Our experience contrasts with these findings [25]. We have observed that persistent subfoveal detachment can also be present after pars plana vitrectomy, although it is more prevalent after scleral buckling surgery. We conducted a prospective study in 48 eyes in 48 patients [4], with primary macula-off RRD and preoperative visual acuity of 20/200 or worse, who underwent successful scleral buckling (SB) surgery (23 patients) and pars plana vitrectomy (PPV) (23 patients). One month postoperatively, 41% in the SB group versus 33% in PPV group had persistent subfoveal fluid on OCT. At the 6-month visit, 12.5% in both groups showed subfoveal fluid. None of the patients had subfoveal fluid at the 24-month follow-up visit. Resolution of subfoveal fluid was not accompanied by a significant increase in final VA in the subgroup of patients with subfoveal fluid (p=0.28; Fig. 11.4).

The functional disorder of the detached retina is thought to be due to the lack of transported material (e.g., photomaterial, glucose, and ions) between the sensory retina and retinal pigment epithelium [5, 16]. Nevertheless, in some studies, visual acuity in eyes with residual subretinal fluid improved to the same degree as that of eyes

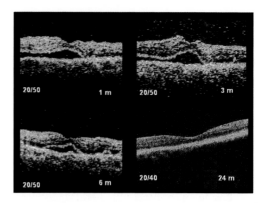

Fig. 11.4 Evolution of a case with postoperative subfoveal fluid after scleral buckling surgery from month 1 to month 24 post-surgery and the changes in visual acuity during follow-up in Snellen lines

with a flat fovea. This improvement suggests that recovery of vision is, to some extent, due to the close proximity of the sensory retina and retinal pigment epithelium even in the presence of a small amount of subretinal fluid. This proximity, resulting from closure of the retinal breaks, might allow intercellular transportation of materials and activation of photoreceptor cells.

References

1. Aylward GW. Optimal procedures for retinal detachments. In: Ryan SJ (2006) Retina. Elsevier Mosby, Los Angeles.

2. Baba T, Hirose A, Moriyama H, Mochizuki M. Tomographic image and visual recovery of acute macula-off rhegmatogenous retinal detachment. Graefes Arch Clin Exp Ophthalmol (2004) 242:576–581.

3. Benson WE, Nantawan P, Morse PH. Characteristics and prognosis of retinal detachments and demarcation lines. Am J Ophthalmol (1977) 84:641–644.

4. Boixadera A, Martinez-Castillo V, Garcia-Arumi J. Two-year optical coherence tomography and visual acuity outcomes after successful repair of acute macula-off retinal detachment. 23rd Meeting of the American Society of Retina Specialists, Montreal, 17/7/05. Oral Communication.

5. Bridges CD, Alvarez RA, Fong SL, Gonzalez-Fernandez F, Lam DMK, Liou GI. Visual cycle in the mammalian eye. Vis Res (1984) 24:1581–1594.

6. Brod RD, Flynn HW, Lightman DA. Asymptomatic rhegmatogenous retinal detachments. Arch Ophthalmol (1995) 113:1030–1032.

7. Byer NE. The natural history of asymptomatic retinal breaks. Ophthalmology (1982) 89:1033–1039.

8. Byer NE. Subclinical retinal detachment resulting from asymptomatic retinal breaks: prognosis for progression and regression. Ophthalmology (2001) 108:1499–1504.

9. Byer NE. Spontaneous regression and disappearance of subclinical rhegmatogenous retinal detachment. Am J Ophthalmol (2001) 131:269–270.

10. Chauhan DS, Marshall J. The interpretation of optical coherence tomography images of the retina. Invest Ophthalmol Vis Sci (1999) 40:2332–2342.

11. Cohen SM. Natural history of asymptomatic clinical retinal detachments. Am J Ophthalmol (2005) 139:777–779.

12. Davis MD, Segal PP, MacCormick A. The natural course followed by the fellow eye in patients with rhegmatogenous retinal detachments. In: Pruett RC, Regan CDJ, eds. Retina Congress. New York: Appleton-Century-Crofts, (1974) pp 643–659.

13. Davis MD. The natural history of retinal breaks without detachment. Trans Am Ophthalmol Soc (1973) 71:343–372.

14. Fercher AF, Hitzenberger CK, Drexler W, Kamp G, Sattmann H. In vivo optical coherence tomography. Am J Ophthalmol (1993) 116:113–114.

15. Folk JC, Sneed SR, Folberg R et al. Early adhesion from laser photocoagulation. Ophthalmol (1989) 96:1523–1525.

16. Glaser BM, Michels RG. Cellular effects of detachment on the neural retina and the retinal pigment epithelium. In: Ryan SJ (ed) Retina. Mosby, St Louis, (1989) pp 165–166..

17. Greven CM, Wall AB, Slusher MM. Anatomic and visual results in asymptomatic clinical rhegmatogenous retinal detachment repaired by scleral buckling. Am J Ophthalmol (1999) 128:618–620.

18. Hagimura N, Suto K, Iida T, Kishi S. Optical coherence tomography of the neurosensory retina in rhegmatogenous retinal detachment. Am J Ophthalmol (2000) 129:186–190.

19. Hagimura N, Iida T, Suto K, Kishi S. Persistent foveal retinal detachment after successful rhegmatogenous retinal detachment surgery. Am J Ophthalmol (2002) 133:516–520.

20. Hee MR, Izatt JA, Swanson EA, Huang D, Schuman JS, Lin CP, Puliafito CA, Fujimoto JG. Optical coherence tomography of the human retina. Arch Ophthalmol (1995) 113:325–332.

21. Hee MR, Baumal CR, Puliafito CA, Duker JS, Reichel E, Wilkins JR, Coker JG, Schuman JS, Swanson EA, Fujimoto JG. Optical coherence tomography of age-related macular degeneration and choroidal neovascularization. Ophthalmology (1996) 103:1260–1270.

22. Hilton GF, Grizzard WS. Pneumatic retinopexy. A two-step outpatient operation without conjunctival incision. Ophthalmology (1986) 93:626–641.

23. Huang D, Swanson EA, Lin CP, Schuman JS, Stinson WG, Chang W, Hee MR, Flotte T, Gregory K, Puliafito CA, Fujimoto JG. Optical coherence tomography. Science (1991) 254:1178–1181.

24. Kishi S, Takahashi H. Three dimensional observations of developing macular holes. Am J Ophthalmol (2000) 130:65–75.

25. Martínez-Castillo V, Boixadera A, Garcia-Arumi J, Corcostegui B. Rate of foveal reattachment. Ophthalmology (2005) 112:947; author reply 947–948.

26. McAllister IL, Meyers SM, Zegarra H, et al. Comparison of pneumatic retinopexy with alternative surgical techniques. Ophthalmology (1988) 95:877–883.

27. Puliafito CA, Hee MR, Lin CP, Reichel E, Schuman JS, Duker JS, Izatt JA, Swanson EA, Fujimoto JG. Imaging of macular disease with optical coherence tomography. Ophthalmology (1995) 102:217–229.

28. Puliafito CA, Hee MR, Schuman JS, Fujimoto JG. Optical coherence tomography of ocular disease. Thorofare, NJ: Slack, (1996) pp 37–288.

29. Schepens CL. Subclinical retinal detachments. Arch Ophthalmol (1952) 47:593–606.

30. Schepens CL. Preventive treatment of idiopathic and secondary retinal detachment. Acta XVIII Concilium Ophthalmologicum Belgica (1958) vol 1:1019–1027.

31. Thompson JT. Discussion on Byer NE. Subclinical retinal detachment resulting from asymptomatic retinal breaks: prognosis for progression and regression. Ophthalmology (2001) 108:1503–1504.

32. Tillery WV, Lucier AC. Round atrophic holes in lattice degeneration. Trans Am Acad Ophthalmol Otolaryngol (1976) 81:509–518.

33. Tolentino FI, Schepens CI, Freeman HM. Vitreoretinal disorders: diagnosis and management. Philadelphia: Saunders (1976) pp 372–399.

34. Tornambe PE, Hilton GF. Pneumatic retinopexy. A multicenter randomized controlled trial comparing pneumatic retinopexy with scleral buckling. The retinal detachment study group. Ophthalmology (1989) 96:772–783.

35. Ung T, Comer MB, Ang AJ, et al. Clinical features and surgical management of retinal detachment secondary to round retinal holes. Eye (2005) 19(6):665–669.

36. Van Effenterre G, Haut J, Larricart P, et al. Gas tamponade as a single technique in the treatment of retinal detachment: is vitrectomy needed? Graefes Arch Clin Exp Ophthalmol (1987) 225:254–258.

37. Wilkins JR, Puliafito CA, Hee MR, Duker JS, Reichel E, Coker JG, Schuman JS, Swanson EA, Fujimoto JG (1996) Characterization of epiretinal membranes using optical coherence tomography. Ophthalmology 103:2142–2151.

38. Wirostko WJ, Han DP, Perkins SL. Complications of pneumatic retinopexy. Curr Opin Ophthalmol (2000) 11:195–200.

39. Wolfensberger TJ. Foveal reattachment after macula-off retinal detachment occurs faster after vitrectomy than after buckle surgery. Ophthalmology (2004) 111:1340–1343.

40. Wolfensberger TJ, Gonvers M. Optical coherence tomography in the evaluation of incomplete visual acuity recovery after macula-off retinal detachments. Graefes Arch Clin Exp Ophthalmol (2002) 240:85–89.

41. Yoon YH, Marmor MF. Rapid enhancement of retinal adhesion by laser photocoagulation. Ophthalmology (1988) 95:1385–1388.

11

Autologous Translocation of the Choroid and RPE in Patients with Geographic Atrophy

12

Antonia M. Joussen, Jan van Meurs, Bernd Kirchhof

Core Messages

- Up till now, there has been no treatment for patients with geographic atrophy.
- Pigment cell transplantation does not prove a long-term benefit in patients with atrophic age-related macular degeneration (AMD).
- Macular rotation surgery may result in the stabilization of vision; however, there are reports of a rapid recurrence of geographic atrophy.
- Translocation of the retinal pigment epithelium and choroid (free graft translocation) has been investigated in patients with neovascular AMD.
- Free graft translocation is feasible in patients with geographic atrophy, leading to reading ability in selected patients.
- Despite a renewed retinal pigment epithelium (RPE) sheet with detectable autofluorescence, areas of decreased sensitivity upon microperimetry do not fully regain function.
- There is still a need for a long-term follow-up with regard to the vitality and functionality of the transplants. Surgical techniques should be refined to reduce the complication profile and to make free graft translocation accessible to a broader group of patients and surgeons.

12.1 Introduction: Pathology and Epidemiology

Non-neovascular age-related macular degeneration (AMD) is characterized by a mostly gradual loss of vision that is associated with drusen, pigment changes, and the development of geographic atrophy. The areas of atrophy tend to succeed the disappearance or flattening of soft drusen, pigment epithelial detachment, or reticular mottling of the retinal pigment epithelium. The atrophic areas continue to enlarge over time, even when already large at initial examination. The combination of reduced visual acuity with enlargement of atrophy, occurring bilaterally in most patients, can lead to significant impairment of visual function [18]. There is intraindividual symmetry in eyes with bilateral geographic atrophy in the presence of a wide range of interindividual variability [2]. Although one can assume that 80% of the patients with neovascular AMD, but only 20% of the patients with dry AMD will reach legal blindness in the affected eye, the total number of patients with dry AMD is five times higher than that for neovascular disease.

Owen and coworkers recently showed that the incidence of severe visual loss from dry AMD is close to the incidence of severe visual loss from exudative AMD [12]. This is reflected by the number of our patients with reading difficulties related to dry AMD.

The pathophysiologic mechanisms underlying the atrophic process, which involves not only the retinal pigment epithelial cells (RPE), but also the outer neurosensory retina and the choriocapillaris, are poorly understood. Atrophy of the retinal pigment epithelium is followed by atrophy of the choriocapillaris [14].

Interestingly, areas of increased fundus autofluorescence outside geographic atrophy may be associated with variable degrees of loss of retinal sensitivity [15] and precede the development and enlargement of outer retinal atrophy in eyes with AMD [5].

12.2   Treatment Approaches in Patients with Geographic Atrophy

While there is currently no pharmacological treatment available to reactivate RPE function, replacement strategies of the diseased RPE become more attractive.

Attempts to replace diseased RPE by autologous IPE cells in suspension did not result in a long-term improvement in visual acuity [10, 11, 19], although a small case series report stated that in non-exudative AMD, RPE suspension transplants showed no evidence of rejection and were associated with the disappearance of drusen [1]. Still, so far no conclusive long-term prevention of retinal and choroidal atrophy from cell transplantation has been demonstrated [22].

Three hundred and sixty degree macular translocation was considered in patients with geographic atrophy as a heroic attempt to halt the degenerative process of the outer retinal layers. Macular translocation creates a more healthy RPE bed by rotating the sensory retina away from an area of damaged RPE to a site with intact RPE and has been reported for the treatment of patients with geographic atrophy [3, 4, 8]. Although all reports demonstrate an initial improvement in distance and near vision, a rapid recurrence of atrophy in the area of the translocated fovea was observed by all groups.

Possibly, the RPE cells in the location of the new fovea are even less equipped to cope with the burden or toxic effect of the foveal photoreceptors than the native foveal RPE [8]. Even more likely, the RPE cells that resemble the neo-macula after 360° macular rotation are close to the original foveal RPE cells and thus may be pre-damaged.

12.3   Concept of Translocation of a Free Choroidal: RPE Graft (Free Graft Translocation)

Peyman et al. first suggested translocation of the peripheral choroid and RPE [13]. Later on, van Meurs demonstrated the clinical feasibility of a free RPE–choroidal graft in a pilot study [3, 20, 21].

We have recently reported on functional and anatomical outcome after free graft translocation in 45 patients, the majority of whom had neovascular AMD [6]. Re-vascularization was observed as early as 3 weeks after surgery. Preoperative distant visual acuity ranged from 20/800 to 20/40. Comprehensive evaluation of reading ability using the Radner test demonstrated reading ability in 31 out of 45 eyes preoperatively. Visual outcome after free graft translocation was unrelated to the type of AMD. Patients without intraoperative or postoperative complications were more likely to present with improved reading ability after 6 months. Fixation on the graft was positively related to visual acuity. In most patients, autofluorescence of the pigment epithelium was coincident with revascularization of the graft. Unfortunately, the intra- and postoperative complication profile was high in this first series and revisional surgery was required in 22 eyes due to proliferative vitreoretinopathy (PVR), retinal detachment, macular pucker, or vitreous hemorrhage. In 8 patients the graft was renewed. Nevertheless, in conclusion, autologous translocation of a full-thickness transplant of the choroid and RPE usually results in a vascularized and functioning graft.

The free graft translocation combines the translocation of a monolayer of the RPE together with the adjacent choroids. Although the theoretical concept is convincing, so far, no detailed experience is available on the feasibility of graft in patients with geographic atrophy.

12.3.1   Patients and Methods

We investigated the functional and anatomical outcome of the peripheral autologous translocation of the choroid and RPE in 12 patients with geographic atrophy and recent loss of reading vision (loss of ability to read newspaper print within the past 3 months) [6].

For the present report only patients with a completed follow-up of 6 months or more were considered. Use of warfarin and other antico-agulants including platelet coagulation inhibitors (nonsteroidal antiphlogistic drugs NSAIDS) such as aspirin was stopped before inclusion in the study. Eligible eyes had best corrected visual acuity (BCVA) corresponding to Snellen fractions of 20/40 to 20/800 (VA scores of 68-3). The study is consistent with the Declaration of Helsinki and was approved by the Ethics Committee of the Medical Faculty of the University of Cologne, Germany. Before inclusion, written informed consent was obtained from each patient. Patients were informed about alternative therapeutic modalities (e.g., rheopheresis and vitamin substitution) and the benefits and expected complications of each treatment.

All eyes were examined prior to surgery (baseline examination) and were follow-up visits were scheduled 6 weeks, 3 months, and 6 months postoperatively.

At each follow-up visit, a protocol refraction, BCVA measurement using Early Treatment Diabetic Retinopathy Study (ETDRS) charts, reading performance using Radner Charts, ophthalmoscopic examination, color fundus photography, autofluorescence measurement, fluorescein and indocyanine green (ICG) angiography, fixation testing, and fundus controlled microperimetry using the scanning laser ophthalmoscope were performed.

12.3.2 Free Graft Translocation Surgery in Dry AMD

The detailed surgical procedure is described elsewhere [7]. In short, a standard three-port pars plana vitrectomy was performed. The central retina was then separated from the RPE by subretinal injection of BSS using a glass pipette close to the vascular arcades. The retinotomy site was enlarged and in all patients but one Bruch's membrane, the choroid, and the RPE were intentionally damaged under the fovea to allow for a later re-vascularization of the transplant through Bruch's membrane. After demarcation

of a rectangular excision area of 4–8 disc diameters in size in the lower mid-periphery outside the vascular arcade, the graft was grasped from the choroidal side and inserted underneath the macula through the retinotomy. A perfluorocarbon–silicone oil exchange (Densiron; Fluoron, Neu-Ulm, Germany) concluded the procedure. After a minimum of 3 months silicone oil was removed.

Summary for the Clinician

- An autologous peripheral full-thickness graft of the RPE, Bruch's membrane, and the choroid was positioned under the macula in patients with geographic atrophy.
- Assessment of anatomic and functional outcomes and determination of postoperative complications were followed up for 6 months. Functional tests included ETDRS distant vision, reading (Radner Test), threshold static perimetry, and determination of the point of fixation using the scanning laser ophthalmoscope (SLO). Fluorescein and ICG angiography, autofluorescence, and optical coherence tomography (OCT) served to evaluate the anatomical outcome.

12.3.3 Results

12.3.3.1 Free Graft Translocation Surgery and Complication Profile

Translocation of a free graft of the RPE and choroid was successfully performed in all patients. Four patients presented with tight retina–RPE adhesion resulting in macular hole formation during hydrodissection in one instance. In one patient a small peripheral retinal tear or dialysis occurred intraoperatively and was treated by cryotherapy or by photocoagulation.

Postoperative complications presented as PVR with retinal detachment in 5 eyes, subretinal hemorrhage in 1 eye, fibrinous reaction in 1 eye after silicone oil removal, failure of re-vascularization in 2 cases, and macular pucker requiring re-operation in 2 cases. Peeling of the ILM was performed in 2 cases at the time of silicone oil removal and in 1 eye during re-operation. In none of these eyes significant fibrosis of the graft occurred. None of the eyes in this series developed choroidal neovascularization in the area of the graft. A detailed list of the complications in each patient is published elsewhere [6].

12.3.3.2 Anatomical Outcome: Funduscopic Appearance, Vascularization, and Autofluorescence of the Graft

Throughout a 6-month follow-up, the area of geographic atrophy remained similar in size and shape. RPE atrophy due to intraoperative damage during the insertion of the graft was present in some eyes, especially in the area of the retinotomy.

As reported in our previous series of free autologous graft of the RPE and choroid after choroidal neovascularization (CNV) extraction, the vascularization pattern of the grafts suggested connection of the choroidal channels of the transplant to those of the underlying recipient choroids [6, 21, 22]. Most patients presented with re-vascularization of the graft as early as 6 weeks after translocation (10 out of 12 patients; Fig. 12.1).

Interestingly, in two patients in whom Bruch's membrane was not intentionally damaged, complete re-vascularization was delayed or absent, and two patients did not show any vascularization (but intact autofluorescence) of the graft during the initial follow-up. In general, eyes that initially demonstrated successful re-vascularization of the graft remained vascularized throughout the 6-month follow-up.

Autofluorescence of the grafts was evaluated comparing mean gray-scale values of the graft with mean values outside the macula [6]. Interestingly, the mean autofluorescence of the RPE on the graft amounted to 84±7% of the

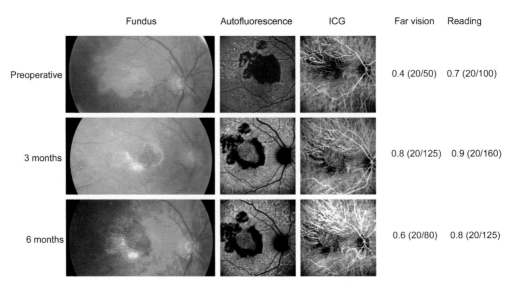

Fig. 12.1 Follow-up of a patient presenting after autologous translocation of the retinal pigment epithelium (RPE) and choroid in geographic atrophy. In this patient geographic atrophy just affected a remaining RPE peninsula. After surgery, visual acuity was stable and reading ability slightly deteriorated, while full vascularization was achieved. Autofluorescence of the graft was present and remained stable during the follow-up. At 6-month follow-up the graft showed good vascularization and both visual acuity and reading vision had significantly improved. *ICG* indocyanine green

autofluorescence of the area outside the macula 6 weeks after surgery, 80±9% 3 months after surgery, and 70±16% at the 6-month follow-up. At this point, autofluorescence of the grafts can be considered stable; however, a long-term follow-up is needed to determine whether the overall intensity decreases significantly over time. There were no areas of RPE atrophy throughout the transplants.

Similar to the series of patients with neovascular AMD [6], vascularization of the graft was not coincident with autofluorescence of the RPE in all cases. While in one case vascularization was missing throughout the follow-up, autofluorescence even remained stable until 1 year after surgery.

Visual acuity did not correlate with intensity of autofluorescence. Similar to our previous observations, there was no difference in central fundus autofluorescence between patients with reading ability and those with worse vision who were unable to read.

12.3.3.3 Functional Outcome: Distant Visual Acuity, Reading Ability, Fixation, and Microperimetry During the Postoperative Course

Three-month (n=11) postoperative vision ranged from 1.6 to 0.5 logMAR (20/800 to 20/50; mean 1.07±0.4 logMAR). Six-month postoperative vision ranged from 2.0 to 0.2 logMAR (hand movements = 20/2,000 to 20/32; mean 0.98±0.6 logMAR; Fig. 12.2). None of the changes was significant. Although patients with initial acuity of ≤0.4 logMAR (20/50 or better) initially deteriorated, they stabilized during the course and even began to improve 3 months after surgery. In contrast, patients with an initial acuity of >1.0 logMAR (<20/200) did not improve in visual acuity during the follow-up. All patients with a 6-month visual acuity of less than 20/200 (logMAR 1.0) suffered postoperative complications. There was a significant visual loss (15 letters or more) in 45% (5 out of 11) of the patients

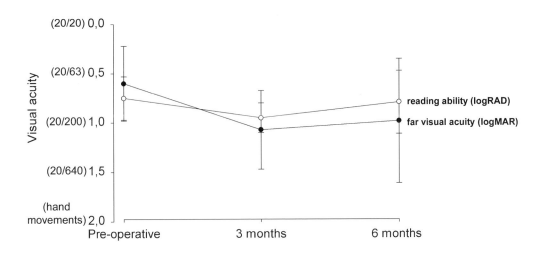

Fig. 12.2 Fundus autofluorescence and fixation after autologous translocation of the RPE and choroid in a patient with geographic atrophy. While this patient demonstrated a predominantly stable fixation on the graft in the initial postoperative phase, there is increasing autofuorescence at the point of fixation 6 months after surgery associated with an improvement in fixation that is likely to be attributable to RPE hyperplasia

3 months after surgery. Interestingly, there were a number of patients who improved or remained stable during the follow-up, resulting in a lower percentage of patients with a significant visual loss at the 6-month follow-up (4 out of 12, 33%). A severe visual loss (30 letters or more) occurred in 27% of the patients (3 out of 11) 3 months after surgery and in only 2 out of 12 eyes (17%) at the 6-month follow-up.

Comprehensive evaluation of reading ability using the Radner test demonstrated reading ability in 9 out of 12 eyes preoperatively. Two of the patients unable to read prior to surgery gained reading ability during follow-up. Two patients lost reading ability due to either intraoperative or postoperative complications. Eight out of 12 patients were able to read at the 6-month follow-up. Overall, reading remained stable throughout the follow-up (Fig. 12.2).

Determination of the mean fixation point (MFP) was achieved during fundus perimetry and confirmed by fixation testing using a moving target (Foerster cross) as described previously [6]. A preoperative stable fixation, even in a small peninsula, resulted in maintenance of this point of fixation after free graft translocation surgery. Stabilization of fixation after free graft translocation was observed in selected patients with initial diffuse fixation.

Fundus microperimetry was performed using a scanning laser ophthalmoscope (SLO; Rodenstock, Munich, Germany). Areas of RPE atrophy associated with lack of autofluorescence presented with absolute scotoma. Small islands of remaining RPE cells were associated with an area of better sensitivity. Figure 12.3 demonstrates a patient with a small peninsula of intact RPE with central fixation preoperatively. Within this peninsula high sensitivity was present. Outside the peninsula a scotoma was found over the RPE atrophy. The newly developed difficulty in reading encountered by this patient may result from the deterioration of this small peninsula. Interestingly, 6 months postoperatively, reading was possible, but the areas of absolute scotomata persisted even though the retina was overlaying the graft, while the good sensitivity of the previous peninsula did not change [7].

12

Summary for the Clinician

- Preoperative visual acuity ranged from 20/800 to 20/40 with a reading vision of 1.1 to 0.5 logRAD. Three patients were unable to read. Two patients without reading ability preoperatively were able to read after surgery. Reading was possible in a total of 8 patients at the 6-month follow-up (1.3 to 0.4 logRAD).
- In all eyes but two, re-vascularization was visible on ICG angiography as early as 3 weeks after surgery.
- Autofluorescence of the pigment epithelium was coincident with re-vascularization of the graft and persisted throughout the follow-up.
- In cases of preoperative fixation on a central RPE peninsula, fixation remained at this position throughout the follow-up.
- Areas overlying atrophic areas demonstrated low threshold sensitivities that persisted after free RPE and choroid grafts with only limited recovery. Areas with preoperatively higher threshold sensitivities maintained their sensitivity throughout the follow-up.
- Recurrent RPE atrophy on the graft was not observed in any of the patients during the short follow-up of 6 months.

12.4 Comment

According to the current hypothesis RPE cell atrophy leads to secondary changes in the choriocapillaris and finally geographic atrophy. Atrophy progresses with time, often sparing the fovea until late in the course of the disease [18]. Importantly, the outer retinal layers are initially not involved and loss of photoreceptors and degeneration of retinal structures only occur later in the course of the disease. Although the nuclei of the outer nuclear layer in eyes with geographic atrophy are markedly attenuated in histological sections, the nuclei of the inner nuclear layer and the ganglion cells remain relatively preserved [9]. This suggests that therapies aimed at replacing outer nuclear function, such as RPE replacement strategies, may be feasible for restoring vision in these patients.

Although it is surgically feasible to transplant fetal RPE to the subretinal space of patients with geographic atrophy, such an allogenic RPE transplant without immunosuppression leads to leakage on fluorescein angiography and eventually to fibrosis. A very weak immune response against proteins associated with photoreceptors is also of concern [22]. The problems associated with cell suspensions and the lack of ability of the trans-

planted cells to form a stable monolayer have been discussed extensively [10, 11, 19].

Interestingly, the rejection rate of human RPE allograft is lower in non-exudative than in neovascular AMD and human RPE allografts are not invariably rejected in the subretinal space without immunosuppression. It seems that an intact blood–retinal barrier is likely to protect against rejection [1].

The free graft technique uses RPE and choroidal tissue from the same patient and thus does

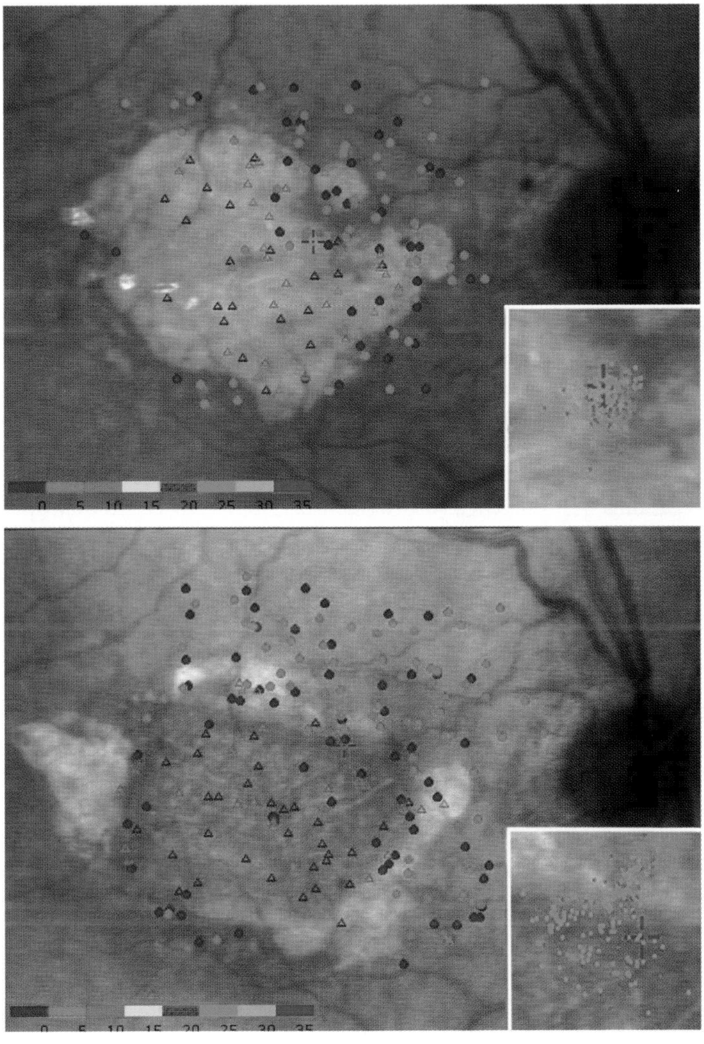

Fig. 12.3 Far vision and reading performance after autologous translocation of the RPE and choroid in patients with geographic atrophy. Preoperative visual acuity and reading performance were assessed throughout a follow-up of 3 months

not carry a risk of rejection. Still, this observation in patients with atrophic AMD seems relevant to our observation in free graft translocation. In free graft translocation, an intact Bruch's membrane leads to a nonperfusion of the graft. While in these patients autofluorescence even remained stable for 1 year, the lack of vascularization was associated with a central scotoma and excentric fixation. Larger groups of patients are required to find out whether vascularization is required for long-term function of the graft.

Taken even further, one could assume that intentional damage of the barrier function of Bruch's membrane would allow for uncontrolled outgrowth of choroidal neovascularization. In our series so far no CNV formation was observed; however, only a long-term follow-up and larger patient series might help to conclude whether the transplanted complex of unaffected choroid and RPE is able to control the subretinal environment. Further studies are then needed to evaluate which humoral factors are involved.

In general, the most relevant question is whether long-term stability and benefit can be achieved with free graft translocation in geographic atrophy. The rapid and early (4–9 months after surgery) recurrence and development of geographic atrophy in the translocated fovea after 360° macular translocation raised new questions regarding the pathogenesis of geographic atrophy [3, 8]. So far it seems that free graft translocation is not associated with the danger of progressing recurrent atrophy, possibly because the transplant is taken from an area of "healthier" RPE distant from the posterior pole of the eye. This is in accordance with what we learned from the first series on free graft translocation in patients with neovascular AMD: no atrophy occurred and RPE autofluorescence remained stable for at least 6 months [6]. Nevertheless, one has to check for pigment mottling or increasing RPE atrophy, even in patients with geographic atrophy.

Fundus controlled perimetry is a precise method of delineating smaller scotomata in the macular area as well as determining parameters of visual function apart from visual acuity. Geographic atrophy and its pathophysiology recently gained scientific interest when autofluorescence in the junctional zone of atrophy was related to function as tested by microperimetry [5]. While

studies indicate that scotopic sensitivity loss exceeds photopic sensitivity loss in patients with geographic AMD [16], SLO-based fundus perimetry, as applied in our study, does not allow for differentiation between photopic or scotopic photoreceptor responses. However, in our current study, autofluorescence demonstrated stable values within the graft area throughout the follow-up with a definite autofluorescence in the graft area compared with a previous lack of autofluorescence throughout the area of atrophy. Interestingly, areas of atrophy that demonstrated a reduced sensitivity prior to surgery generally did not recover, even though autofluorescence was re-established by the graft. Limited plasticity was seen in islets with remaining high sensitivities. Enlargement of these areas allowed reading vision in selected patients. Thus, one can summarize that autofluorescence might be a relevant measure in the extension of existing lesions [5, 16]; however, this does not allow a predictive statement with regard to free graft translocation. From our study it seems impossible to draw a conclusion regarding function from the autofluorescence of the underlying graft once a degenerative process of the disease has resulted in changes in the retina.

Furthermore, this means that graft translocation in patients with geographic atrophy, if meant to improve vision, is dependent on early treatment when central retinal function is still present. In our series, patients with diffuse initial fixation, indicating a long-standing degenerative process, regained neither stable fixation postoperatively nor functional improvement as determined by microperimetry.

Even though the technical feasibility of free graft translocation had been demonstrated previously [6, 17, 20, 21], we still encountered a high postoperative complication rate.

At this stage we can conclude that free graft translocation in patients with geographic atrophy stabilizes macular functions in most patients and can rarely improve reading vision. The procedure, however, is tarnished by surgical and postoperative complications. Refinement of the surgical procedures may affect the complication rate in the future and may determine whether this approach can become the treatment of choice for patients with geographic atrophy. Furthermore, additional knowledge about the significance of autofluorescence in these patients is required. However, if further studies confirm that free graft translocation does prevent recurrent RPE atrophy, this treatment might not only be beneficial for the patients, but also revitalize discussions on the pathophysiology of dry AMD.

Summary for the Clinician

- The translocation of a full-thickness graft usually results in a vascularized and functioning graft in patients with geographic atrophy.
- A longer follow-up is necessary to learn about the long-term survival and functionality of the graft.

Acknowledgements

The authors acknowledge Sandra Joeres, MD; Florian Heussen, BS; and Nader Fawzy, BS for excellent patient follow-up.

References

1. Algvere PV, Berglin L, Gouras P, Sheng Y, Kopp ED. Transplantation of RPE in age-related macular degeneration: observations in disciform lesions and dry RPE atrophy. Graefes Arch Clin Exp Ophthalmol 1997;235:149–158.

2. Bellmann C, Jorzik J, Spital G, Unnebrink K, Pauleikhoff D, Holz FG. Symmetry of bilateral lesions in geographic atrophy in patients with age-related macular degeneration. Arch Ophthalmol 2002;120:579–584.

3. Cahill MT, Mruthyunjaya P, Bowes Rickman C, Toth CA. Recurrence of retinal pigment epithelial changes after macular translocation with 360 degrees peripheral retinectomy for geographic atrophy. Arch Ophthalmol 2005;123:935–938.

4. Eckardt C, Eckardt U. Macular translocation in non-exudative age-related macular degeneration. Retina 2002;22:786–794.

5. Holz FG, Bellman C, Staudt S, Schütt F, Völcker HE. Fundus autofluorescence and development of geographic atrophy in age-related macular degeneration. Invest Ophthalmol Vis Sci 2001;42:1051–1056.

6. Joussen AM, Heussen FMA, Joeres S, Llacer H, Prinz B, Rohrschneider K, Maaijwee KJM, van Meurs J, Kirchhof B. Autologous translocation of the choroid and RPE in age related macular degeneration. Am J Ophthalmol 2006;142:17–30.

7. Joussen AM, Joeres S, Fawzy N, Heussen FMA, Llacer H, van Meurs J, Kirchhof B. Autologous translocation of the choroid and RPE in patients with geographic atrophy. Ophthalmology, accepted for publication.

8. Khurana RN, Fujii GY, Walsh AC, Humayun MS, de Juan E Jr, Sadda SR. Rapid recurrence of geographic atrophy after full macular translocation for nonexudative age-related macular degeneration. Ophthalmology 2005;112:1586–1591.

9. Kim SY, Sadda S, Humayun MS, de Juan E Jr, Melia BM, Green WR. Morphometric analysis of the macula in eyes with geographic atrophy due to age-related macular degeneration. Retina 2002;22:464–470.

10. Lappas A, Weinberger AWA, Foerster AMH, Kube T, Kirchhof B. Iris pigment epithelium translocation in age related macular degeneration. Graefes Arch Exp Clin Ophthalmol 2000;238:631–641.

11. Lappas A, Foerster AM, Weinberger AW, Coburger S, Schrage NF, Kirchhof B. Translocation of iris pigment epithelium in patients with exudative age-related macular degeneration: long-term results. Graefes Arch Clin Exp Ophthalmol 2004;242:638–647.

12. Owen CG, Fletcher AE, Donoghue M, Rudnicka AR. How big is the burden of visual loss caused by age related macular degeneration in the United Kingdom? Br J Ophthalmol 2003;87:312–317.

13. Peyman GA, Blinder KJ, Paris CJ, Alturki W, Nelson NC, Desai U. A technique for retinal pigment epithelium transplantation for age-related macular degeneration secondary to extensive subfoveal scarring. Ophthalmic Surg 1991;22:102.

14. Schatz H, Mc Donald R. Atrophic macular degeneration: rate of spread of geographic atrophy and visual loss. Ophthalmology 1989;96:1541–1551.

15. Schmitz-Valckenberg S, Bultmann S, Dreyhaupt J, Bindewald A, Holz FG, Rohrschneider K. Fundus autofluorescence and fundus perimetry in the junctional zone of geographic atrophy in patients with age-related macular degeneration. Invest Ophthalmol Vis Sci 2004;45:4470–4476.

16. Scholl HP, Bellmann C, Dandekar SS, Bird AC, Fitzke FW. Photopic and scotopic fine matrix mapping of retinal areas of increased fundus autofluorescence in patients with age-related maculopathy. Invest Ophthalmol Vis Sci 2004;45:574–583.

17. Stanga PE, Kychenthal A, Fitzke FW, Halfyard AS, Chan R, Bird AC, Aylward GW. Retinal pigment epithelium translocation after choroidal neovascular membrane removal in age-related macular degeneration. Ophthalmology 2002;109:1492–1498.

18. Sunness JS, Gonzales-Baron J, Applegate CA, et al. Enlargement of atrophy and visual acuity loss in the geographic atrophy form of age-related macular degeneration. Ophthalmology 1999;106:1768–1779.

19. Thumann G, Aisenbrey S, Schraermeyer U, et al. Transplantation of autologous iris pigment epithelium after removal of choroidal neovascular membranes. Arch Ophthalmol 2000;118:1350–1355.

20. Van Meurs JC. Retinal pigment epithelium and choroid translocation in patients with exudative age-related macular degeneration. In: Kirchhof B, Wong D (eds) Essentials of ophthalmology: vitreoretinal surgery. Springer, Berlin Heidelberg New York, 2005; pp 73–87.

21. Van Meurs JC, Van Den Biesen PR. Autologous retinal pigment epithelium and choroid translocation in patients with exudative age-related macular degeneration: short-term follow-up. Am J Ophthalmol 2003;136:688–695.

22. Weisz JM, Humayun MS, De Juan E Jr, Del Cerro M, Sunness JS, Dagnelie G, Soylu M, Rizzo L, Nussenblatt RB. Allogenic fetal retinal pigment epithelial cell transplant in a patient with geographic atrophy. Retina 1999;19:540–545.

Subject Index